T0318647

NETosis

NETosis
Immunity, Pathogenesis and Therapeutics

Geeta Rai
Associate Professor, Department of Molecular
and Human Genetics, Institute of Science,
Banaras Hindu University, Varanasi, Uttar Pradesh, India

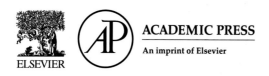

ACADEMIC PRESS
An imprint of Elsevier

ELSEVIER

Notices
Knowledge and best practice in this field are constantly changing. As new research and experience broaden
our understanding, changes in research methods, professional practices, or medical treatment may become
necessary.

Practitioners and researchers must always rely on their own experience and knowledge in evaluating and
using any information, methods, compounds, or experiments described herein. In using such information or
methods they should be mindful of their own safety and the safety of others, including parties for whom they
have a professional responsibility.

To the fullest extent of the law, neither the Publisher nor the authors, contributors, or editors, assume any
liability for any injury and/or damage to persons or property as a matter of products liability, negligence or
otherwise, or from any use or operation of any methods, products, instructions, or ideas contained in the
material herein.

British Library Cataloguing-in-Publication Data
A catalogue record for this book is available from the British Library

Library of Congress Cataloging-in-Publication Data
A catalog record for this book is available from the Library of Congress

ISBN: 978-0-12-816147-0

For Information on all Academic Press publications
visit our website at https://www.elsevier.com/books-and-journals

Publisher: Andre Gerhard Wolff
Acquisition Editor: Glyn Jones
Editorial Project Manager: Sam Young
Production Project Manager: Sreejith Viswanathan
Cover Designer: Christian Bilbow

Typeset by MPS Limited, Chennai, India

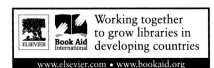

Working together
to grow libraries in
developing countries

www.elsevier.com • www.bookaid.org

In the loving memory of Mummy

Contents

Foreword

Our understanding of neutrophil biology and its role in microbial clearance, immune regulation, and disease pathology has advanced outstandingly in recent years. In the past decade, several new aspects of neutrophil functions have emerged, instituting their significance not only in microbial defense in the host but also in impacting many pathological consequences. Neutrophil extracellular traps (NETs) which are a network of chromatin structures have been at the core of this renewed interest in neutrophil research. Recognition of NET inducing triggers and molecules that modulate NET formation has conferred imperative relevance to the role of NETs in immune protection, and various diseases including inflammatory, autoimmune diseases, and cancer.

Progress in NETosis-related research has greatly improved our understanding of its role in immunological processes and diseases. Recent studies have recognized NETs to be a source of inflammatory mediators and autoantigens, which when released during NETosis serve to activate immune cells and cytokines which further stimulate NETosis. Blocking the process of NETosis or inhibiting the activity of components in NETs might be effective in the treatment of diseases and resolving inflammation. There is a promising prospect for the evolution of novel pharmacological interventions based on knowledge of the process of NETosis and the interplay of NET components and the immune system.

NETosis although is currently intensively investigated yet, due to the enormous complexity of the process, many aspects on the regulation and role of NETosis are not well perceived and therefore a systematic review and assemblage of information on this topic is sought exceedingly. Therefore the purpose of this book is to present and discuss the current knowledge about the mechanisms of NETosis and its role in the regulation of immune response and the pathogenesis of various diseases. This book has come at a time when NET biology is assuming global dimensions in research, life science/medical education, and training. This may be observed that the author in this well laid out book has compiled key findings and concepts that have thus far accumulated and shaped the field of NET biology.

Furthermore to state, the main objective of this book, therefore, is to provide the readers with relevant information as a base on which to build a superior understanding of NETosis. I am happy to note that this book has been well structured and designed to adequately meet the research/curriculum requirements in life sciences and medicine. The book will serve as a source of reference for immunologists, academicians, research scientists, pharmaceutical sector, and postgraduate and undergraduate students. Summarily, it may be observed that this publication is an outcome of sincere and dedicated efforts made by the author who deserves to be appreciated for compiling various aspects of NETosis and I am sure this book will be a highly useful addition to NETosis literature.

Prof. Rakesh Bhatnagar
Vice Chancellor, Banaras Hindu University, Varanasi, India
January 2019

Preface

Immunology is a rapidly growing field of science and with continuous developments of new concepts in all wings including cellular, humoral, innate, and adaptive immunology. The profoundness of the assimilated knowledge achieved from immunological research on various mechanisms of immunity has always had an impact on the medical practices. One such interesting dynamic process which caught much attention and interest of immunologists globally, around a decade ago was "Neutrophil extracellular trap formation" also referred as "NETosis." It is described as a unique antimicrobial process originally discovered in neutrophils which involves chromatin decondensation and degranulation leading to the formation of a NET-like structure that entraps and neutralizes microbes. Research interest of immunologists in this process in the past few years has soared tremendously resulting in the emergence of various new concepts on the variants of the mechanism, triggers, signaling molecules and pathways, its implications on a variety of diseases and pathologies, and a new direction of NET-based therapy. NETosis research outcomes have resulted in an accumulation of knowledge so vast that a pressing need for a book was felt that could integrate and compile an assemblage of the available information. The mechanism of NET formation continues to fascinate scientists and researchers and the emergence of newer concepts is enriching the understanding of the molecular and cellular mechanisms of the NETosis. Yet due to enormous complexity of the process many aspects on the regulation and function remain less understood.

The book "NETosis: Immunity, Pathogenesis and Therapeutics," has been written with an emphasis on understanding the fundamental process of NETosis and integrating into its framework the latest research in the field. This book includes a wide array of topics ranging from introduction and basic concepts of this dynamic process, molecular mechanisms and signaling, antimicrobial strategies adopted, regulatory factors, status of NETosis in newborns, in autoimmunity, and other diseases to emergence of NET-based therapeutics. This book is an attempt to provide detailed and updated research on various aspects of the process deemed necessary for complete comprehension and assimilation of the existing knowledge for translation into medical practices.

As a sole author writing each chapter from information congregated from more than 100 reference papers (per chapter) had been an arduous and enormously testing experience but the fact that it helped preserve uniformity of style and approach in the whole book without breaking the flow of information is a significant gain.

The book is composed of six chapters. The first chapter on introduction of NET formation describes the process and the sequence of events involved. Description of distinct forms of NETosis has been provided along with mechanisms of clearance and regulation, and concludes with an account of this process operative in other cells like basophils, eosinophils, mast cells, and monocytes. The second chapter elaborates on the role of DNA and proteins involved in NETosis. Details of signaling pathways known till date and role of kinases have been discussed. This chapter also provides an understanding of antimicrobial strategies adopted by the cells for different microbes like bacteria, viruses, fungi, and parasites along with relevance of cytokines in NETosis. The third chapter focuses on how different factors regulate this process. NETosis is discussed in the context of other cell death pathways like autophagy, apoptosis, and necrosis to show how it discerns from them and yet there are common interphases. Various triggers involved and the impact of hypoxic condition and pH has also been discussed in relation to NET formation.

The fourth chapter builds on the elucidation of the distinct status of this process in pregnancy and newborns. Inhibitory factors and differential regulation of NET components existing in newborns have been discussed. In the fifth chapter the role of NETosis in contributing to the autoantigen pool and eventually inciting autoimmunity has been discussed. NET components play a major role in induction of autoimmune disease like rheumatoid arthritis, systemic lupus erythematosus, and multiple sclerosis. In addition, the chapter elaborates on the emergence of a new line of NET-based therapeutics that has the potential for management of autoimmune diseases. The sixth and the final chapter provides a detailed description on the role of NETosis and its components in a host of other diseases like cystic fibrosis, diabetes mellitus, cardiometabolic disease, cancer, Alzheimer's, gout, pancreatic, and infectious diseases. In this chapter different NET-based therapeutic approaches being used or proposed have been discussed. To allow better comprehension for the readers each chapter has been integrated with illustrations created and designed in tune with the concepts built in each chapter.

The author is of strong understanding that the elaborated details on several aspects of the process would be of immense use to students, academicians, and researchers in all major fields of life sciences like immunology, medicine, cell biology, biochemistry, and genetics and hope that the knowledge and research outcomes assimilated in this book would help not only to boost advanced research but would also facilitate bench to bedside translation.

Finally, I would like to thank and acknowledge all those who have made a significant contribution and supported me in my journey of writing this book. It is with great pleasure I would like to acknowledge my students Doli Das, Sakshi Singh, Khusbu Priya, and Hirak Jyoti Das for their invaluable assistance in the preparation of this book. They also helped create visually appealing figures from my rough layouts and sketches. I also acknowledge the cooperation of my laboratory manager, Sudhanshu Rai, for sharing the responsibilities of the laboratory that allowed me to focus on my book writing. I express gratitude and appreciation to my family friends Sangeeta and Dr. Pradeep Srivastava for their support. I am thankful to my family members Dr. Samarjit Singh, Shailja, Vivek, Devrat, Harshita, Skand, and Pooja for their encouragement and forbearance. I owe a lot to my father Mr. Awadhesh Kumar Rai and my mother Late Mrs. Prem Lata Rai for shaping the course of my life. My beautiful kids Shambhavi and Arnav have been my sweet stressbusters and a source of boundless joy and love. My husband Dr. Rajesh Kumar needs a special mention not only for his love and care but also for his immense support in providing high quality input and critical insights for this book.

Geeta Rai

Chapter 1

Neutrophil extracellular trap formation: an introduction

Neutrophils are the immune cells characterized by a lobulated nucleus, earning them the designation of polymorphonuclear cells (PMNs). Attributed by the abundance of granules in their cytoplasm and their staining with neutral dyes, Paul Ehrlich first called these cells as neutrophils during the 19th century. When the immune system is under a challenge from pathogens, neutrophils are the first cells to exit the circulation and relocate to the area under attack. Through their antimicrobial activity, neutrophils kill microbes, communicate the damage status to other immune cells by releasing small signaling molecules, and initiate healing. With an arsenal of potent antimicrobial proteins at their disposal, neutrophils are the professional phagocytes that, together with the production of reactive oxygen species (ROS), kill microbes inside the phagosome. Through "degranulation," these antimicrobial proteins are also released. Armed with broadly effective antimicrobials that are stored predominately in specialized granules, neutrophils are the most abundant innate immune effector cells of the human immune system. A third antimicrobial mechanism is the release of neutrophil extracellular traps (NETs). First noticed by Takei et al. (1996), as a unique form of cell death, distinct from necrosis or apoptosis neutrophils were found to kill bacteria by forming extracellular structures called NETs, which are composed mainly of DNA, histones, and proteases, such as neutrophil elastase (NE). This process was further studied and termed as NETosis in 2004 (Brinkmann et al., 2004). In NETosis the neutrophils upon induction of innate immune sensors with pathogenic antigens extrude large amounts of chromatin and granule proteins, such as NE and myeloperoxidase (MPO), which trap and kill microorganisms. NETs contain the invading microorganism to prevent the spread of infection and use their highly localized arsenal of antimicrobial peptides to neutralize and kill the microorganism. With its ability to damage host tissues, neutrophil arsenal deploys itself in a tightly regulated manner during the release of NETs (Brinkmann et al., 2004).

NETosis. DOI: https://doi.org/10.1016/B978-0-12-816147-0.00001-0

Two distinct forms of NETosis

Current process of NET release follows a bimodal approach. According to the first model, NETosis is a cell death pathway of chromatin decondensation, nuclear and cytoplasmic membrane disintegration followed by the expulsion of the chromatin and granular contents into the extracellular space (Brinkmann et al., 2004, 2007; Fuchs et al., 2010). In contrast to apoptotic cells, neutrophils undergoing NETosis do not appear to display phosphatidylserine and other "eat me" signals, which might prevent their silent clearance by phagocytes. NET disassembly takes place primarily by nucleases (Fuchs et al., 2007).

The second model involves ejection of DNA/serine proteases from intact neutrophils, and also mitochondrial DNA release that works by activating inflammation and is apparently not associated to cell death (Yousefi, Mihalache, Kozlowski, Schmid, & Simon, 2009). In addition to these, autophagy may also contribute to NETosis (Remijsen, Berghe, & Wirawan, 2011).

Suicidal NETosis

Conventional suicidal NETosis is triggered by engagement of IgG−Fc receptors, Toll-like receptors, complement, or cytokines on neutrophils (Brinkmann et al., 2004; Garcia Romo et al., 2011; Munks et al., 2010). These receptors once activated initiates the downstream cascade, wherein calcium sequestered inside endoplasmic reticulum is released as calcium ions into the cytoplasm (Fig. 1.1). This elevation of calcium levels in the cytoplasm increases the activity of protein kinase C (PKC) and phosphorylation of gp91phox, heme binding subunit of the superoxide-generating NADPH oxidase (Kaplan et al., 2012). This initiates the assembly of the subunits of NADPH oxidase in the cytosol and bounds to the membrane into functional complexes at cytoplasmic or phagosomal membranes (also called phagocytic oxidase, PHOX) and the successive generation of ROS (Papayannopoulos, Metzler, Hakkim, & Zychlinsky, 2010). ROS causes rupture of granules and nuclear envelope, and eventually fusing of released nuclear, granular, and cytoplasmic contents occurs. NE (a serine protease of broad specificity) and MPO (peroxidase enzymes that produce antimicrobial hypohalous acids), usually stored in azurophilic granules, move to the nucleus. Subsequently, NE breaks down the linker histone H1 and processes the core histones and MPO which augment chromatin decondensation causing the release of extracellular traps (ETs) (Papayannopoulos et al., 2010). NE also degrades actin cytoskeleton, blocking phagocytosis of neutrophils. Another important enzyme, peptidyl arginine deiminase type 4 (PAD4), causes deamination of histones and their proteolytic cleavage initiated before nuclear breakdown additionally contributes to chromatin decondensation (Pingxin et al., 2010; Saskia, John, Sanja, & Kerra, 2011). The breakdown of the plasma

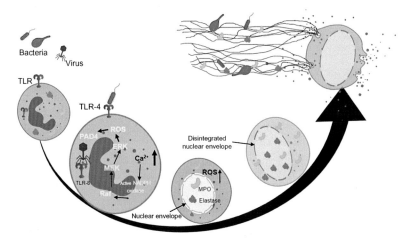

FIGURE 1.1   Suicidal NETosis. Inducer/stimuli bind to endogenous and exogenous receptors. Raf/MEK/ERK kinases pathway activation leading to increase in cytosolic calcium leads to phosphorylation of gp91phox protein. This activates the NADPH oxidase complex and subsequently produces reactive oxygen species (ROS). Elastase and myeloperoxidase then translocate to the nucleus stimulated by ROS and other yet unknown factors. The chromatin decondenses that result in the loss of lobular shape of the nucleus. Loss of nuclear envelope and granular membrane takes place and decondensed chromatin is associated with cytoplasmic components. Plasma membrane is lost and DNA is released as extracellular traps.

membrane releases NETs and NET-entrapping pathogens, resulting in cell death with loss of viable cell functions like migration and phagocytosis also referred to as beneficial suicide (Papayannopoulos et al., 2010).

Vital NETosis

As opposed to the conventional form of NETosis, Clark et al. (2007) in a straight forward experiment reported that release of NEs from neutrophils continued without penetration of intracellular DNA staining dye SYTOX Green, emphasizing the fact that neutrophils remain structurally intact. This was evidence for a first alternative pathway of NETosis and the authors coined the term vital NETosis to refer it (Fig. 1.2). This was further supported by electron microscopy images of *Staphylococcus aureus*—induced NETs which are formed by blebbing of the nuclear envelope and vesicular exportation in vitro and in vivo (Bianchi et al., 2009). Similar catapult, like the release of mitochondrial DNA without lytic cell rupture, has been first reported by Yousefi and colleagues in eosinophils, but subsequently in neutrophils (Yousefi, Gold, & Andina, 2008; Yousefi et al., 2009). Contrary to this, a new report described the formation of eosinophil extracellular trap (EET) resulting in cytolytic granular release (Ueki et al., 2013). Thus, granulocytes, in general, may have both a lytic and a nonlytic pathway of NETosis.

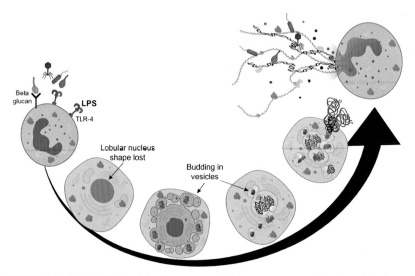

FIGURE 1.2 Vital NETosis. Stimuli are recognized by receptors on cell surface. Lobular and multinucleated shape of the nucleus is lost. External and internal nuclear membranes are lost and budding of vesicles takes place. Pearl strings form of DNA filaments are formed inside vesicles in the cytoplasm, dense cytoplasmic granules approach towards intact plasma membrane. DNA is released as extracellular traps through a small area in the cell surface; some cytoplasmic granules also fuse with plasma membrane that is released into extracellular space to associate with DNA.

Differences between suicidal and vital NETosis

The main differences between suicidal NETosis and vital NETosis depend on the nature of inciting stimuli and NET release programming mechanism and requires hours of stimulation for extracellular trap formation. For example, suicidal NETosis has mostly been established in the context of phorbol-12-myristate-13-acetate (PMA)−induced chemical stimulation and requires hours. In contrast, vital NETosis has been exhibited to be activated by microbial-specific molecular patterns called as pathogen-associated molecular patterns (PAMPs) or endogenous damage-associated molecular patterns (DAMPs) recognized by host pattern recognition receptors. One such PAMP is, bacterial lipopolysaccharide (LPS), a Gram-negative bacterial stimulus, which causes rapid NET release without the involvement of cell lysis and was precisely mediated by toll-like receptor 4 (TLR4) in platelets that assisted activation of neutrophils. In addition, enactment of the vital NETosis pathway has all the earmarks of being a summed up reaction against different classes of microbial pathogens. Likewise, *S. aureus* prompts human neutrophils to quickly discharge NETs by means of nuclear envelope blebbing and vesicular exportation, in this manner preserving PMN plasma membrane integrity. In vivo, TLR-2 and complement (Yipp, Petri, & Salina, 2012) mediate rapid release of NETs following infection by live Gram-positive bacteria. Besides, recent reports suggest NETosis indeed takes place rapidly within 30 minutes upon stimulation with *Candida albicans* in fibronectin- and complement-dependent manner. A second significant contrast between vital NETosis and conventional suicidal NETosis varies with the working capacity of the neutrophils during NET release. As reported by early in vitro findings, microbe-induced NETosis liberated the neutrophils from lysis maintaining the functional capacity of the NETosing neutrophils. Kolaczkowska et al. (2015) in their laboratory used intravital confocal microscopy to develop a method for directly visualizing NETosis in a mouse model of a bacterial skin infection. They demonstrated that within the skin, neutrophils rapidly eject NETs in a TLR-2- and complement-mediated pathway while maintaining the proficiency of chemotaxing and phagocytosing live bacteria. Amid the underlying acute reaction neither PMN lysis nor confirmation of cell death was clear; in any case, NETosing neutrophils progressed toward becoming nuclear cytoplasts fit for pursuing and detaining live *Staphylococcus* (Yipp et al., 2012).

The third essential distinction among suicidal NETosis and vital NETosis composed of the components utilized to make and discharge NETs. Suicidal NETosis necessitates PMA stimulation of Raf-MEK-ERK and consequent activation of NADPH oxidase (Hakkim et al., 2011). The decondensation of chromatin is facilitated by MPO and elastase ensuing in a mixture of DNA and granule proteins that are extruded out of a perforation in the plasma membrane. In comparison, vital NETosis requires trafficking of DNA within vesicles from the nucleus to the extracellular space.

NETosis: sequence of events

NET formation from reactive oxygen species to chromatin decondensation

ROS-mediated pathway of NETosis requires two enzymes. NADPH oxidase which generates ROS and stimulates MPO, triggering activation and translocation of NE packed in azurophilic granules to the nucleus, wherein chromatin packaging is disrupted by proteolytic cleavage of histones by NE (Fig. 1.3). This allows MPO to bind to the chromatin and assists NE in enzyme-independent decondensation of chromatin (Papayannopoulos et al., 2010). However, NADPH oxidase activity is not exclusive, as mitochondrial ROS generated by immune complexes is sufficient to drive NETosis (Lood et al., 2016). Azurophilic granules release NE without membrane rupture or fusion. This is mediated by azurosome, a complex in resting neutrophils spanning granule membranes where a fraction of MPO is bound to NE (Metzler, Goosmann, Lubojemska, Zychlinsky, & Papayannopoulos, 2014). Hydrogen peroxide selectively releases NE into the cytosol in an

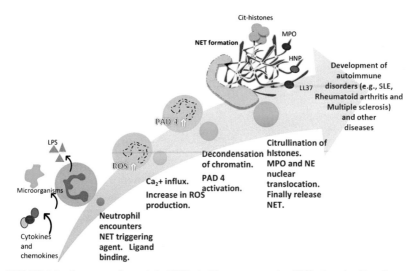

FIGURE 1.3 Sequence of events in NETosis. Upon encountering NET triggering ligands, neutrophils undergo increased calcium influx and reactive oxygen species (ROS) generation. This leads to activation of protein-arginine deiminase 4 (PAD4) activation and subsequent chromatin decondensation due to histone citrullination of human nuclear proteins (HNPs). In addition, myeloperoxidase (MPO) and neutrophil elastase (NE) contributes further to the decondensation process, finally releasing NETs. NETs further contribute to development of autoimmune diseases and other pathologies.

MPO-dependent manner. MPO enzymatic inhibition does not block but only delays NETosis as evident from experiments (Metzler et al., 2011), possibly owing to activation of proteolytic activity of NE against large protein substrates mediated by MPO. This oxidative activation facilitates NE binding to F-actin filaments in the cytoplasm, degrading them in order to enter the nucleus (Metzler et al., 2014). Although NE is sufficient to decondense nuclei in vitro (Papayannopoulos et al., 2010), disassembly of the nuclear envelope in neutrophils may be assisted by unknown mechanisms. Several NET stimuli such as fungi and crystals also induce this MPO−NE pathway (Schauer et al., 2014; Warnatsch, Ioannou, Wang, & Papayannopoulos, 2015). Its role is further supported by studies of neutrophils from patients with chronic granulomatous disease (CGD) (Fuchs et al., 2007) and with complete MPO deficiency (Metzler et al., 2011), as well as by studies using NE-deficient mice or NE inhibitors in mouse models of sepsis, cancer, and pulmonary infection (Branzk et al., 2014; Cools-Lartigue et al., 2013; Kolaczkowska et al., 2015; Papayannopoulos et al., 2010). NADPH oxidase−deficient mice also demonstrate abrogated NET release during pulmonary fungal infection, which otherwise stimulates robust NET release (Rohm et al., 2014). Similarly, cysteine protease cathepsin C (CTSC) is also involved in NETosis as it is defective in neutrophils from patients with

Papillon–Lefèvre syndrome caused by mutations in the protein, which processes NE into its mature form (Roberts, 2016; Sorensen et al., 2014). Another protein DEK that is involved in nuclear chromatin binding has recently been implicated in NETosis as DEK-deficient neutrophils exhibit defective NETosis and can be rescued by addition of exogenous recombinant DEK protein, which suggests that DEK binding promotes chromatin decondensation in a similar manner to MPO (Mor-Vaknin et al., 2017).

Histone modification in NETosis

Histone modifications such as deamination or citrullination contribute to chromatin decondensation driven by protein-arginine deiminase type 4 (PAD4), an arginine citrullinating nuclear enzyme that acitrullinates arginine residues, converting amine groups to ketones (Wang et al., 2004). In spite of evidence supporting requirement of a reducing activity for PAD4 activity, inhibition of NADPH oxidase decreases citrullination. Moreover, PAD4 can be sufficiently activated by hydrogen peroxide (Li et al., 2010; Neeli, Dwivedi, Khan, & Radic, 2009), which requires calcium (Vossenaar et al., 2004) and is activated by PKCζ (Neeli and Radic, 2013), a kinase that is implicated in the ROS burst. Altogether, these observations imply PAD4 lies downstream of ROS and calcium signaling during NETosis.

Histone citrullination during NETosis is also induced by physiological stimuli such as fungi and crystals (Branzk et al., 2014; Warnatsch et al., 2015). However, chromatin decondensation as a contributor has been more difficult to assess (Leshner et al., 2012; Li et al., 2010; Wang et al., 2010). Experiments with PAD4 inhibition in cell lines or with mouse neutrophils derived from PAD4-deficient mice were first difficult to infer owing to low NET yields (Lewis et al., 2015; Li et al., 2010). One of the complications is that histone citrullination is often used as the sole marker to detect NETs in PAD4-deficient or PAD4-inhibited mice (Knight et al., 2014; Wong et al., 2015). Whether NE activity is exclusive for histone citrullination to promote chromatin decondensation is unclear. Chromatin decondensation is blocked by NE inhibitors during pulmonary fungal infection without interfering with histone H3 citrullination (Branzk et al., 2014), which suggests that histone citrullination occurs independently of NE activity, although it might not be sufficient to drive chromatin decondensation. Recent findings suggest that the list of citrullinated proteins in NETosis induced by microorganisms or PMA is dominated by histones and is distinct from extensive protein hyper-citrullination associated with stress inducers such as ionomycin, pore-forming toxins, and immune complexes (Romero et al., 2013; Knight et al., 2014). Therefore different NET-inducing stimuli might engage PAD enzymes in diverse ways, and the pattern of citrullinated substrates could help to determine the relevant immunopathogenic mechanisms in vivo.

Mechanism of clearance of NETotic debris

The mechanisms for clearance of NETs after their disposal are less well understood. During infection, NETs persist for several days (Branzk et al., 2014) and are thought to be dismantled by the secreted plasma nuclease DNase I (Hakkim et al., 2010). Injection of this enzyme during *S. aureus* infection leads to rapid degradation of NET-associated DNA, but the dynamics of NET clearance by endogenous enzymes are unknown. Strikingly, NET proteins persist long after DNA degradation (Kolaczkowska et al., 2015), suggesting that there are additional clearance mechanisms that might involve macrophage scavenging, as DNase I facilitates the ingestion of NETs by macrophages in vitro (Farrera & Fadeel, 2013).

Regulation of NETosis

NETs neutralize and kill bacteria (Brinkmann et al., 2004), fungi (Urban, Reichard, Brinkmann, & Zychlinsky, 2006), viruses (Saitoh et al., 2012), and parasites (Abi Abdallah et al., 2012) and are thought to prevent bacterial and fungal disseminations (Branzk et al., 2014; Walker et al., 2007). However, dysregulated NETs can contribute to the pathogenesis of immune-related diseases, so NETosis must be tightly regulated to prevent any pathology. The microorganism size is one of numerous factors that influence NETosis. The sensing of pathogen size depends on the competition for NE access between NETosis and phagocytosis. This mechanism enables deployment of NETs in neutrophils against large microorganisms. Small microorganisms sequester NE away from the nucleus and blocks chromatin decondensation (Branzk et al., 2014) taken up into phagosomes that fuse with azurophilic granules. The lack of phagosomes in neutrophils combat microorganisms that are excessively large to be devoured allows NE to translocate to the nucleus via the slower azurosome pathway and to drive NETosis. Additionally, release of NE into the cytosol encourages actin cytoskeleton degradation, blocking phagocytosis and committing cells to NETosis (Metzler et al., 2014). The particle size effect on NETosis also pertains to sterile stimuli. Larger, needle-shaped urate crystals trigger NETosis more effectively than urate microaggregates that are small enough to be ingested (Pieterse, Rother, Yanginlar, Hilbrands, & van der Vlag, 2016). This discerning induction of NETosis bounds redundant tissue damage during infection by pathogens that are trivial enough to be killed intracellularly. Accordingly, mice lacking the antifungal phagocytic receptor dectin 1 are incapable to selectively restrain NETosis and are liable to NET-mediated pathology in reaction to small microorganisms. It is possible that NETosis is retained for small virulent microorganisms that impede phagosomal killing. Consistent with this idea, virulent enteropathogenic bacteria induce NET formation, whereas nonvirulent probiotic bacteria do not. One strategy for small microorganisms to elude phagocytosis is aggregation. Large aggregates of *Mycobacterium bovis* Bacillus Calmette—Guérin drive NETosis in a microorganism size-dependent manner (Branzk et al., 2014). On the other hand, microbial intrusion with phagosome maturation may also enable small microorganisms to induce NETosis. *Neisseria gonorrhoeae* delays the fusion of the phagosome with azurophilic granules and induces NETosis (Johnson & Criss, 2013). Virulence mechanisms are also involved in the ability of *P. aeruginosa* to induce NETosis, which depends on expression of a motile flagellum (Floyd et al., 2016). Bacteria that lack flagella fail to elicit a potent ROS burst and NETosis, but flagella alone are not sufficient to induce NETosis. These findings appear to contradict the size-dependence principle.

Several discoveries suggest fluctuating neutrophil cell biology affects microbial virulence factors during NETosis (Yoo, 2014). Many virulent *S. aureus* serotypes kill neutrophils (Spaan, Surewaard, Nijland, & van Strijp, 2013) and might promote the association of NET components by physical lysis of cellular membranes. For example, the *S. aureus* pore-forming toxin, leukotoxin GH, is sufficient to drive NETosis, but it is unclear whether it is required for NET induction by bacteria (Malachowa, Kobayashi, Freedman, Dorward, & DeLeo, 2013). Moreover, expression of invasin, an adhesin that binds β-integrins, potentiates the ROS burst to induce NETosis in response to *Yersinia pseudotuberculosis* (Gillenius & Urban, 2015). Finally, the observation of *Porphyromonas gingivalis* mutants that lack a phagocytosis-promoting protease drive NETosis (Jayaprakash, Demirel, Khalaf, & Bengtsson, 2015) is also consistent with the ability of phagocytosis to regulate NETosis (Wang et al., 2014).

Although NETs were discovered in 2004 (Brinkmann et al., 2004), but we still have limited knowledge on how the formation of NETs is controlled. Induction of isolated neutrophils by PMA is directed to the novel observation that neutrophils form NETs. PMA propels assembly of the multicomponent NADPH oxidase and triggers the production of ROS. The role of oxidant production is observed by studies of neutrophils from patients with CGD, which cannot generate ROS. CGD neutrophils fail to release NETs after exposure to PMA or challenge with *S. aureus*. Disintegration of the nuclear envelope is a distinct hallmark of neutrophils forming NETs (Fuchs et al., 2007) much like nuclear membrane breakdown during cell-cycle progression. Interestingly, recent work observed that activation of cyclin-dependent kinases (CDKs) is critically involved in signaling that leads to NET formation (Amulic, Knackstedt, & Abu, 2017). Silencing of CDK4 and CDK6 abrogates the release of NETs, whereas ROS generation, phagocytosis, and degranulation are not affected. Thus signals driving NET formation resemble cell-cycle signaling, rather than signaling cascades that lead to other types of cell death. However, more evidence is needed to confirm how neutrophils respond to activation of CDK4/6 with cell death rather than cell proliferation. Indeed, whether neutrophils are still viable when they release NETs is a matter of ongoing discussion. Moreover, in separate studies, other groups have challenged the source of NET-DNA, and described that NETs can be formed with mitochondria-derived DNA. This observation was confirmed by recent work linking the immunogenicity of NETs to oxidized DNA of mitochondrial origin (Lood et al., 2016). Suicidal NET formation happens after exposure to high doses of PMA requiring hours of exposure and oxidant generation.

Other cells involved in NETosis

Although ET formation has been intensely described in the context of neutrophils, but it has also been observed in numerous cell types such as macrophages, basophils, eosinophils, and mast cells (MCs). Regardless of the types of cells from which they are released, several features are common in ETs which composed of a DNA backbone decorated with antimicrobial peptides, proteases, and histones; all capable of killing a wide spectrum of microbes (Brinkmann et al., 2004; Fuchs et al., 2007; Urban & Zychlinsky, 2007; von Kockritz-Blickwede & Nizet, 2009). Nevertheless, they also display distinctive differences such as the DNA backbone deriving sub-cellular compartments which may be nucleus or mitochondria, the fraction of reacting cells within the pool, and the molecular mechanism/s triggering ET formation.

The intracellular signaling pathway implicated in ET formation composed of simultaneous generation of reactive oxygen radicals by the activation of NADPH oxidase (Papayannopoulos et al., 2010; Guimaraes-Costa, Nascimento, Wardini, Pinto-da-Silva, & Saraiva, 2012). Several reports also demonstrate that eosinophils and neutrophils release mitochondrial DNA in addition to chromosomal DNA (Yousefi et al., 2008, 2009) to form ETs without induction of cell death. However, its mechanism(s) remain unknown. While ETs primarily function through their antimicrobial effect, its overall role in defense against pathogens is debatable.

Basophils

Due to their pro-inflammatory and immunoregulatory properties, basophils are mostly linked to allergic and parasitic infections. Of late studies have shown the binding of basophils to various bacteria with and without opsonizing antibodies. As shown by Morshed et al. (2014), basophils from both human and mouse are able to form extracellular DNA traps by production of mitochondrial ROS. This is achieved by priming of IL-3 followed by activation of complement factor 5α receptor or FCγRI. Such basophil extracellular traps (BETs) mostly composed of mitochondrial DNA but not nuclear DNA, along with granular proteins such as basogranulin and mouse mast cell protease. Formation of BETs ensues regardless of any operative NADPH oxidase in basophils. The in vivo inflammatory role of BETs is evident from various studies that show BETs can be found in both human and mouse inflamed tissues. In total, these findings are suggestive of direct innate immune effector functions exerted by basophils in the extracellular space (Yousefi et al., 2015).

Eosinophils

Similar to BETs, EETs (Fig. 1.4) are also seen in multiple infectious, allergic, and autoimmune eosinophilic diseases. These EETs comprise a meshwork of DNA fibers embedded with eosinophil granule proteins, such as major basic protein (MBP) and eosinophil cationic protein (ECP). Fascinatingly, EETs also contain mitochondrial DNA in its traps rather than nuclear DNA and might have its origin in the mitochondria. These mitochondrial DNA−ejected eosinophils were still viable as they showed no evidence of a reduced life span. Eosinophils engage multiple activation mechanisms, whereby transmembrane signal transduction processes are initiated by toll-like receptors, cytokine, chemokine, and adhesion receptors leading to the formation of EETs. Eosinophil DNA release also requires the activation of the NADPH oxidase as one of its vital signaling event. EET's involvement has been demonstrated in multiple infectious diseases like spirochetosis, in

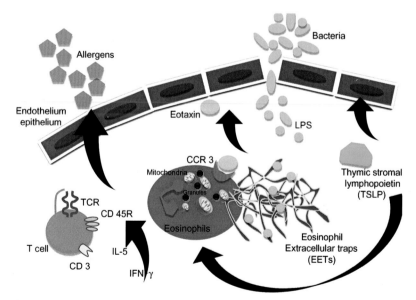

FIGURE 1.4   Extracellular trap formation in eosinophil. Invading bacteria and/or cytokines generated by epithelial cell and/or T-cells might directly activate eosinophils. Cytokine priming with IL-5 or IFN-γ and subsequent stimulation with bacterial LPS, eostaxin or complement factor C5a generates eosinophil extracellular traps (EETs). Adherent eosinophils are also stimulated by thymic stromal lymphopoietin. EETs contain mitochondrial DNA and granule proteins, but no cytosolic, mitochondrial, nuclear or membrane proteins.

which extracellular DNA binds to bacteria as seen in vivo. EETs were also evident in tissues infected with Schistosoma, in infectious skin diseases such as creeping disease and scabies. Eosinophils also exert a protective role in experimental sepsis associated with EETs. EETs are primarily involved in allergic inflammatory diseases such as bronchial asthma, atopic dermatitis, contact dermatitis, and allergic drug reactions. For these implications, future research on EETs has possibilities of yielding novel biomarkers and therapeutic targets in eosinophilic diseases.

Mast cells

Mast cell extracellular traps (MCETs), similar to NETs, are able to entrap and kill various microbes. MCs form MCETs by releasing their nuclear DNA. At the time of allergic reactions and parasitic infections, these MCs play an important part and even essential element of the early host innate immune response to bacterial and fungal pathogens. MCs are involved in the commencement of the early immune response by recruiting neutrophils and macrophages by locally releasing some inflammatory mediators. MCs form MCETs similar to that of professional phagocytes and remove microbes by intracellular as well as extracellular antimicrobial mechanisms. During cellular disintegration, there is release of DNA and some granule proteins which are not the reasons for MCET's formation rather this is a controlled process via specific stimulation and also plays an important role in innate host defense. Extensive number of different mechanisms has been developed by MCs to deal with the invaders and undesirable endogenic factors. These include the synthesis, consequent release and storage of inflammatory mediators that form MCETs and phagocytosis.

Monocytes and macrophages

Macrophages carry out different functions that include tissue repair, regulate homeostasis, and immune function. ETs are formed in response to various microorganisms by macrophages. These ETs formed by monocytes and macrophages are similar to that of the NET's features. The cell death program by which Macrophage extracellular trap (METs) are produced is METosis in which there is release of fibers composed of DNA and studded with cellular proteins. METs along with immobilization and death of some microorganisms also play a part in disease pathology. Like NETs, METs are extracellular fibers composed of DNA that extend outside the cell and are degraded by treatment with DNase I or micrococcal nuclease. In the METs produced by human peripheral blood monocytes and THP-1 macrophage-like cells, there is presence of known ET components such as histones, elastase, or MPO (Halder et al., 2016; Je, Quan, Yoon, Na, Kim, & Seok, 2016).

In 2016 Halder et al. established that the METs released by monocyte can be boosted or increased in the presence of human serum. And also showed that complement factors, C3b and C5b-9, were deposited onto METs when the media-containing serum was infected with *C. albicans*. They suggested that activated complement might add microbicidal activity and allows for the enhanced opsonization and phagocytosis of organisms within ETs during the resolution of inflammatory responses.

Some studies have evaluated the viability of monocyte and macrophage undergoing METosis. In 2010 Chow et al. stained cells for intracellular esterase activity and plasma membrane integrity and found that staining of MET-producing RAW 264.7 macrophage-like cells was steady with a loss of membrane integrity, indicating that these cells were no longer viable. A similar approach was used by Vega et al. (2014) and found that within 3 hours mouse J774A.1 macrophage-like cells producing METs were dead. TUNEL staining of M1-polarized THP-1 cells were done by Nakazawa et al. (2016), to assess these cells releasing extracellular DNA after exposure to NETs. Cells were positive for TUNEL staining which is in contradiction with a report on neutrophils which showed that NET-producing cells are TUNEL negative.

Webster et al. (2010) evaluated the role of caspase-1 in mitosis. They demonstrated that human peripheral blood monocytes infected with either *Escherichia coli* or *Klebsiella pneumonia* resulted in caspase-1 activation, which is a part of pyroptosis, a nonapoptotic cell death pathway. Release of MET decreased with the inhibition of caspase-1 by the chemical Z-YVAD-FMK. During the first 12 hours of infection, they showed loss of cell viability with caspase-1 activation. Earlier caspase-1 was not found to be activated in NETosis whereas it is activated in macrophages in response to NET material and the antibacterial protein, LL-37, present on NET fibers (Kahlenberg, Carmona-Rivera, Smith, & Kaplan, 2013).

The sparse data available suggest that METosis is indeed a cell death process, similar to the classic pathways in neutrophils. More work is needed to define the principal triggers and pathways that move a macrophage from other immune responses to METosis. Additional studies are also needed to differentiate the markers of different cellular death pathways, including METosis, and to clarify the conflicting data.

References

Amulic, B., Knackstedt, S. L., & Abu, A. U. (2017). Cell-cycle proteins control production of neutrophil extracellular traps. *Developmental Cell*, *43*(449-462), e5.

Bianchi, M., Hakkim, A., Brinkmann, V., Siler, U., Seger, R. A., & Zychlinsky, A. (2009). Restoration of NET formation by gene therapy in CGD controls aspergillosis. *Blood, 114*, 2619–2622. Available from https://doi.org/10.1182/blood-2009-05-221606.

Branzk, N., Lubojemska, A., Hardison, S. E., Wang, Q., Gutierrez, M. G., Brown, G. D., & Papayannopoulos, V. N. (2014). Neutrophils sense microbe size and selectively release neutrophil extracellular traps in response to large pathogens. *Nature Immunology, 15*, 1017–1025.

Brinkmann, V., & Zychlinsky, A. (2007). Beneficial suicide: why neutrophils die to make NETs. *Nature Review Microbiology, 5*(8), 577−582. Available from https://doi.org/10.1038/nrmicro1710.

Brinkmann, V., Reichard, U., Goosmann, C., Fauler, B., Uhlemann, Y., & Weiss, D. S. (2004). Neutrophil extracellular traps kill bacteria. *Science, 303*, 1532−1535. Available from https://doi.org/10.1126/science.1092385.

Clark, S. R., Ma, A. C., Tavener, S. A., McDonald, B., Goodarzi, Z., Kelly, M. M., ... Kubes, P. (2007). Platelet TLR4 activates neutrophil extracellular traps to ensnare bacteria in septic blood. *Nature Medicine, 13*, 463469.

Cools-Lartigue, J., Spicer, J., McDonald, B., Gowing, S., Chow, S., Giannias, B., ... Ferri, L. J. (2013). Neutrophil extracellular traps sequester circulating tumor cells and promote metastasis. *Journal of Clinical Investigation, 123*, 3446−3458.

Farrera, C., & Fadeel, B. (2013). Macrophage clearance of neutrophil extracellular traps is a silent process. *Journalof Immunology, 191*, 2647−2656.

Floyd, M., Winn, M., Cullen, C., Sil, P., Chassaing, B., Yoo, D. G., ... Floyd, M. (2016). Swimming motility mediates the formation of neutrophil extracellular traps induced by flagellated Pseudomonas aeruginosa. *Public Library of Science Pathogy, 12*, e1005987.

Fuchs, T. A., Abed, U., Goosmann, C., Hurwitz, R., Schulze, I., Wahn, V., ... AFuchs, T. A. (2007). Novel cell death program leads to neutrophil extracellular traps. *Journal of Cell Biology, 176*, 231−241.

Fuchs, T. A., Brill, A., Duerschmied, D., Schatzberg, D., Monestier, M., & Myers, D. D., Jr. (2010). Extracellular DNA traps promote thrombosis. *Proceeding of National Academy of Science USA, 107*, 15880−15885. Available from https://doi.org/10.1073/pnas.1005743107.

Garcia Romo, G. S., Caielli, S., Vega, B., Connolly, J., Allantaz, F., Xu, Z., ... Pascual, V. (2011). Netting neutrophils are major inducers of type I IFN production in pediatric systemic lupus erythematosus. *Science Translational Medicine, 2*, 73−20.

Gillenius, E., & Urban, C. F. (2015). The adhesive protein invasin of Yersinia pseudotuberculosis induces neutrophil extracellular traps via beta1 integrins. *Microbes and Infection, 17*, 327−336. Available from https://doi.org/10.1016/j.micinf.2014.12.01.

Guimaraes-Costa, A. B., Nascimento, M. T., Wardini, A. B., Pinto-da-Silva, L. H., & Saraiva, E. (2012). METosis: a microbicidal mechanism beyond cell death. *Journal of Parasitology Research, Guzman, 929743*, 2012.

Hakkim, A., Fürnrohr, B. G., Amann, K., Laube, B., Abed, U. A., Brinkmann, V., Herrmann, M., ... Hakkim, A. (2010). Impairment of neutrophil extracellular trap degradation is associated with lupus nephritis. *Proceeding of National Academy of Science USA, 107*, 9813−9818.

Hakkim, A., Fuchs, T. A., Martinez, N. E., Hess, S., Prinz, H., Zychlinsky, A., & Waldmann, H. (2011). Activation of the Raf-MEK-ERK pathway is required for neutrophil extracellular trap formation. *Nature Chemical Biology, 7*, 75−77.

Halder, L. D., Abdelfatah, M. A., Jo, E. A., Jacobsen, I. D., Westermann, M., Beyersdorf, N., ... Skerka, C. (2016). Factor H binds to extracellular DNA traps released from human blood monocytes in response to Candida albicans. *Front Immunology, 7*, 671.

Jayaprakash, K., Demirel, I., Khalaf, H., & Bengtsson, T. (2015). The role of phagocytosis, oxidative burst and neutrophil extracellular traps in the interaction between neutrophils and the periodontal pathogen Porphyromonas gingivalis. *Molecular Oral Microbiology, 30*, 361−375.

Je, S., Quan, H., Yoon, Y., Na, Y., Kim, B. J., & Seok, S. H. (2016). Mycobacterium massiliense induces macrophage extracellular traps with facilitating bacterial growth. *PLoS One, 11*, e0155685.

Johnson, M. B., & Criss, A. K. (2013). Neisseria gonorrhoeae phagosomes delay fusion with primary granules to enhance bacterial survival inside human neutrophils. *Cell Microbiology, 15*, 1323–1340.

Kahlenberg, J. M., Carmona-Rivera, C., Smith, C. K., & Kaplan, M. J. (2013). Neutrophil extracellular trap-associated protein activation of the NLRP3 inflammasome is enhanced in lupus macrophages. *Journal of Immunology, 190*, 1217–1226.

Knight, J. S., Luo, W., O'Dell, A. A., Yalavarthi, S., Zhao, W., ... Kaplan, M. J. (2014). Peptidylarginine deiminase inhibition reduces vascular damage and modulates innate immune responses in murine models of atherosclerosis. *Circulation Research, 114*, 947–956.

Kolaczkowska, E., Jenne, C. N., Surewaard, B. G., Thanabalasuriar, A., Lee, W. Y., Sanz, M. J., Mowen, K., ... Kubes, P. (2015). Molecular mechanisms of NET formation and degradation revealed by intravital imaging in the liver vasculature. *Nature Communication, 6*, 6673.

Leshner, M., Wang, S., Lewis, C., Zheng, H., Chen, X. A., Santy, L., ... Wang, Y. (2012). PAD4 mediated histone hypercitrullination induces heterochromatin decondensation and chromatin unfolding to form neutrophil extracellular trap-like structures. *Frontiers in Immunology, 3*, 307.

Lewis, H. D., Liddle, J., Coote, J. E., Atkinson, S. J., Barker, M. D., Bax, B. D., ... Wilson, D. M. (2015). Inhibition of PAD4 activity is sufficient to disrupt mouse and human NET formation. *Nature Chemical Biology, 11*, 189–191.

Li, P., Li, M., Lindberg, M. R., Kennett, M. J., Xiong, N., & Wang, Y. (2010). PAD4 is essential for antibacterial innate immunity mediated by neutrophil extracellular traps. *Journal of Experimental Medicine, 207*, 1853–1862.

Lood, C., Blanco, L. P., Purmalek, M. M., Carmona-Rivera, C., Ravin, S. S. D., Smith, C. K., ... Kaplan, M. J. (2016). Neutrophil extracellular traps enriched in oxidized mitochondrial DNA are interferogenic and contribute to lupus-like disease. *Nature Medicine, 22*, 146–153.

Malachowa, N., Kobayashi, S. D., Freedman, B., Dorward, D. W., & DeLeo, F. R. (2013). Staphylococcus aureus leukotoxin GH promotes formation of neutrophil extracellular traps. *Journal of Immunology, 191*, 6022–6029.

Metzler, K. D., Fuchs, T. A., Nauseef, W. M., Reumaux, D., Roesler, J., Schulze, I., ... Metzler, K. D. (2011). Myeloperoxidase is required for neutrophil extracellular trap formation: implications for innate immunity. *Blood, 117*, 953–959.

Metzler, K. D., Goosmann, C., Lubojemska, A., Zychlinsky, A., & Papayannopoulos, V. (2014). A myeloperoxidase-containing complex regulates neutrophil elastase release and actin dynamics during NETosis. *Cell Reports, 8*, 883–896.

Morshed, M., Hlushchuk, R., Simon, D., Walls, A. F., Obata-Ninomiya, K., Karasuyama, H., ... Yousefi, S. (2014). *Journal of Immunology, 192*, 5314–5323.

Mor-Vaknin, N., Saha, A., Legendre, M., Carmona-Rivera, C., Amin, M. A., ... Markovitz, D. M. N. (2017). DEK-targeting DNA aptamers as therapeutics for inflammatory arthritis. *Nature Communication, 8*, 14252.

Munks, M. W., McKee, A. S., Macleod, M. K., Powell, R. L., Degen, J. L., & Reisdorph, N. A. (2010). Aluminum adjuvants elicit fbrin-dependent extracellular traps in vivo. *Blood, 116* (24), 5191–5199. Available from https://doi.org/10.1182/blood-2010-03-275529.

Nakazawa, D., Shida, H., Kusunoki, Y., Miyoshi, A., Nishio, S., Tomaru, U., ... Ishizu, A. (2016). The responses of macrophages in interaction with neutrophils that undergo NETosis. *Journal of Autoimmunity, 67*, 19–28.

Neeli, I., Dwivedi, N., Khan, S., & Radic, M. (2009). Regulation of extracellular chromatin release from neutrophils. *Journal of Innate Immunity, 1*, 194–201.

Neeli, I., & Radic, M. (2013). Opposition between PKC isoforms regulates histone deimination and neutrophil extracellular chromatin release. *Frontiers in Immunology, 4*, 38.

Papayannopoulos, V., Metzler, K. D., Hakkim, A., & Zychlinsky, A. (2010). Neutrophil elastase and myeloperoxidase regulate the formation of neutrophil extracellular traps. *Journal of Cell Biology, 191*, 677−691.

Pieterse, E., Rother, N., Yanginlar, C., Hilbrands, L. B., & van der Vlag, J. (2016). Neutrophils discriminate between lipopolysaccharides of different bacterial sources and selectively release neutrophil extracellular traps. *Frontiers in Immunology, 7*, 484. Available from https://doi.org/10.3389/fmmu.2016.00484.

Pingxin, I., Ming, I., Lindberg, M. R., Kennett, M. J., Na, X., & Yanming, W. (2010). PAD4 is essential for antibacterial innate immunity mediated by neutrophil extracellular traps. *Journal of Experimental Medicine, 207*(9), 1853−1862. Available from https://doi.org/ 10.1084/jem.20100239.

Remijsen, Q., Berghe, T. V., & Wirawan, E. (2011). Neutrophil extracellular trap cell death requires both autophagy and superoxide generation. *Cell Research, 21*, 290−304.

Roberts, H. (2016). Characterization of neutrophil function in Papillon-Lefevre syndrome. *Journal of Leukocyte Biology, 100*, 433−444.

Rohm, M., Grimm, M. J., DAuria, A. C., Almyroudis, N. G., Segal, B. H., & Urban, C. F. (2014). NADPH oxidase promotes neutrophil extracellular trap formation in pulmonary aspergillosis. *Infection and Immunity, 82*, 1766−1777. Available from https://doi.org/ 10.1128/IAI.00096-14.

Romero, V., Fert-Bober, J., Nigrovic, P. A., Darrah, E., Haque, U. J., Lee, D. M., . . . Romero, V. (2013). Immune-mediated pore-forming pathways induce cellular hypercitrullination and generate citrullinated autoantigens in rheumatoid arthritis. *Science Translational Medicine, 5*, 209ra150.

Saitoh, T., Komano, J., Saitoh, Y., Misawa, T., Takahama, M., Kozaki, T., . . . Akira, S. (2012). Neutrophil extracellular traps mediate a host defense response to human immunodeficiency virus-1. *Cell Host Microbe, 12*, 109−116. Available from https://doi.org/10.1016/j. chom.2012.05.015.

Saskia, H., John, R. T., Sanja, A., & Kerra, A. M. (2011). PAD4-mediated neutrophil extracellular trap formation is not required for immunity against influenza infection. *PLoS One, 6*(7), e22043. Available from https://doi.org/10.1371/journal.pone.0022043.

Schauer, C., Janko, C., Munoz, L. E., Zhao, Y., Kienhöfer, D., Frey, B., . . . Schauer, C. (2014). Aggregated neutrophil extracellular traps limit inflammation by degrading cytokines and chemokines. *Nature Medicine, 20*, 511−517.

Sorensen, O. E., et al. (2014). Papillon-Lefevre syndrome patient reveals species-dependent requirements for neutrophil defenses. *Journal of Clinical Investigation, 124*, 4539−4548.

Spaan, A. N., Surewaard, B. G., Nijland, R., & van Strijp, J. A. (2013). Neutrophils vs *Staphylococcus aureus*: A biological tug of war. *Annual Review of Microbiology, 67*, 629−650.

Takei, H., Araki, A., Watanabe, H., Ichinose, A., & Sendo, F. (1996). Rapid killing of human neutrophils by the potent activator phorbol 12-myristate 13-acetate (PMA) accompanied by changes different from typical apoptosis or necrosis. *Journal of leukocyte biology, 59*, 229−240.

Ueki, S., Melo, R. C., Ghiran, I., Spencer, L. A., Dvorak, A. M., & Weller, P. F. (2013). Eosinophil extracellular DNA trap cell death mediates lytic release of free secretion-competent eosinophil granules in humans. *Blood, 121*(11), 2074−2083.

Urban, C., & Zychlinsky, A. (2007). Netting bacteria in sepsis. *Nature Medicine*, *13*, 403−404.

Urban, C. F., Reichard, U., Brinkmann, V., & Zychlinsky, A. (2006). Neutrophil extracellular traps capture and kill *Candida albicans* yeast and hyphal forms. *Cellular Microbiology*, *8* (4), 668−676. Available from https://doi.org/10.1111/j.1462-5822.2005.00659.

Vega, V. L., Crotty Alexander, L. E., Charles, W., Hwang, J. H., Nizet, V., & De Maio, A. (2014). Activation of the stress response in macrophages alters the M1/M2 balance by enhancing bacterial killing and IL-10 expression. *Journal of Molecular Medicine, (Berl)*, *92*, 1305−1317.

Von Kockritz-Blickwede, M., & Nizet, V. (2009). Innate immunity turned inside-out: antimicrobial defense by phagocyte extracellular traps. *Journal of Molecular Medicine*, *87*, 775−783.

Vossenaar, E. R., Radstake, T. R., Van der Heijden, A., Van Mansum, M. A., Dieteren, C., De Rooij, D. J., . . . Van Venrooij, W. J. (2004). Expression and activity of citrullinating peptidylarginine deiminase enzymes in monocytes and macrophages. *Annals of The Rheumatic Diseases*, *63*, 373−381.

Walker, M. J., et al. (2007). DNase Sda1 provides selection pressure for a switch to invasive group A streptococcal infection. *Nature Medicine*, *13*, 981−985.

Wang, Y. (2004). Human PAD4 regulates histone arginine methylation levels via demethylimination. *Science*, *306*, 279−283.

Wang, Y. (2010). Histone hypercitrullination mediates chromatin decondensation and neutrophil extracellular trap formation. *Journal of Cell Biology*, *184*, 205−213.

Wang, Y. (2014). Increased neutrophil elastase and proteinase 3 and augmented NETosis are closely associated with beta-cell autoimmunity in patients with type 1 diabetes. *Diabetes*, *63*, 4239−4248.

Warnatsch, A. A., Ioannou, M., Wang, Q., & Papayannopoulos, V. (2015). Inflammation. Neutrophil extracellular traps license macrophages for cytokine production in atherosclerosis. *Science*, *349*, 316−332.

Webster, S. J., Daigneault, M., Bewley, M. A., Preston, J. A., Marriott, H. M., Walmsley, S. R., . . . Dockrell, D. H. (2010). Distinct cell death programs in monocytes regulate innate responses following challenge with common causes of invasive bacterial disease. *Journal of Immunology*, *185*, 2968−2979.

Wong, S. L. (2015). Diabetes primes neutrophils to undergo NETosis, which impairs wound healing. *Nature Medicine*, *21*, 815−819.

Yipp, B. G., Petri, B., & Salina, D. (2012). Infection induced NETosis is a dynamic process involving neutrophil multitasking in vivo. *Nature Medicine*, *18*(9), 1386−1393.

Yoo, D. G. (2014). Release of cystic fibrosis airway inflammatory markers from *Pseudomonas aeruginosa*-stimulated human neutrophils involves NADPH oxidase-dependent extracellular DNA trap formation. *Journal of Immunology*, *192*, 4728−4738.

Yousefi, S., Gold, J. A., & Andina, N. (2008). Catapult-like release of mitochondrial DNA by eosinophils contributes to antibacterial defense. *Nature Medicine*, *14*(9), 949−953.

Yousefi, S., Mihalache, C., Kozlowski, E., Schmid, I., & Simon, H. U. (2009). Viable neutrophils release mitochondrial DNA to form neutrophil extracellular traps. *Cell Death and Differentiation*, *16*(11), 1438−1444.

Yousefi, S., Morshed, M., Amini, P., Stojkov, D., Simon, D., von Gunten, S., . . . Simon, H. U. (2015). Basophils exhibit antibacterial activity through extracellular trap formation. *Allergy*, *70*, 1184−1188. Available from https://doi.org/10.1111/all.12662.

Further reading

Mayer, F. L., Wilson, D., & Hube, B. (2013). *Candida albicans* pathogenicity mechanisms. *Virulence*, *4*, 119−128. Available from https://doi.org/10.4161/viru.22913.

Mitroulis, I., Kambas, K., Chrysanthopoulou, A., Skendros, P., Apostolidou, E., Kourtzelis, I., ... Ritis, K. (2011). Neutrophil extracellular trap formation is associated with IL-1beta and autophagy-related signaling in gout. *PLoS One*, *6*, e29318.

Mollerherm, H., Neumann, A., Schilcher, K., Blodkamp, S., Zeitouni, N. E., & Dersch, P. (2015). *Yersinia enterocolitica*-mediated degradation of neutrophil extracellular traps (NETs). *FEMS Microbiology Letters*, *362*, fnv192. Available from https://doi.org/10.1093/femsle/fnv192.

Moorthy, A. N., Narasaraju, T., Rai, P., Perumalsamy, R., Tan, K. B., & Wang, S. (2013). In vivo and in vitro studies on the roles of neutrophil extracellular traps during secondary pneumococcal pneumonia after primary pulmonary influenza infection. *Frontiers in Immunology*, *4*, 56. Available from https://doi.org/10.3389/fmmu.2013.00056.

Moorthy, A. N., Rai, P., Jiao, H., Wang, S., Tan, K. B., & Qin, L. (2016). Capsules of virulent pneumococcal serotypes enhance formation of neutrophil extracellular traps during in vivo pathogenesis of pneumonia. *Oncotarget*, *7*, 19327−19340. Available from https://doi.org/10.18632/oncotarget.8451.

Moreno-Altamirano, M. M., Rodriguez-Espinosa, O., Rojas-Espinosa, O., PliegoRivero, B., & Sanchez-Garcia, F. J. (2015). Dengue virus serotype-2 interferes with the formation of neutrophil extracellular traps. *Intervirology*, *58*, 250−259. Available from https://doi.org/10.1159/000440723.

Mulcahy, H., Charron-Mazenod, L., & Lewenza, S. (2008). Extracellular DNA chelates cations and induces antibiotic resistance in *Pseudomonas aeruginosa* biofilms. *PLoS Pathogens*, *4*, e1000213. Available from https://doi.org/10.1371/journal.ppat.1000213.

Nathan, C. (2006). Neutrophils and immunity: Challenges and opportunities. *Nature Reviews Immunology*, *6*, 173−182. Available from https://doi.org/10.1038/nri1785.

Neeli, I., Khan, S. N., & Radic, M. (2008). Histone deimination as a response to inflammatory stimuli in neutrophils. *Journal of Immunology*, *180*, 1895−1902.

Netea, M. G., Joosten, L. A., van der Meer, J. W., Kullberg, B. J., & van de Veerdonk, F. L. (2015). Immune defence against Candida fungal infections. *Nature Reviews Immunology*, *15*, 630−642. Available from https://doi.org/10.1038/nri3897.

Neumann, A., Berends, E. T., Nerlich, A., Molhoek, E. M., Gallo, R. L., & Meerloo, T. (2014). The antimicrobial peptide LL-37 facilitates the formation of neutrophil extracellular traps. *Biochemical Journal*, *464*, 3−11. Available from https://doi.org/10.1042/BJ20140778.

Nusrat, A., von Eichel-Streiber, C., Turner, J. R., Verkade, P., Madara, J. L., & Parkos, C. A. (2001). Clostridium difficile toxins disrupt epithelial barrier function by altering membrane microdomain localization of tight junction proteins. *Infection and Immunity*, *69*, 1329−1336. Available from https://doi.org/10.1128/IAI.69.3.1329-1336.2001.

Oehmcke, S., Morgelin, M., & Herwald, H. (2009). Activation of the human contact system on neutrophil extracellular traps. *Journal of Innate Immunity*, *1*, 225−230.

Paape, M. J., Bannerman, D. D., Zhao, X., & Lee, J. W. (2003). The bovine neutrophil: Structure and function in blood and milk. *Veterinary Research*, *34*, 597−627.

Pacello, F., Ceci, P., Ammendola, S., Pasquali, P., Chiancone, E., & Battistoni, A. (2008). Periplasmic Cu,Zn superoxide dismutase and cytoplasmic Dps concur in protecting *Salmonella enterica* serovar Typhimurium from extracellular reactive oxygen species. *Biochimica et Biophysica Acta*, *1780*, 226−232. Available from https://doi.org/10.1016/j.bbagen.2007.12.001.

Palmer, L. J., Cooper, P. R., Ling, M. R., Wright, H. J., Huissoon, A., & Chapple, I. L. (2012). Hypochlorous acid regulates neutrophil extracellular trap release in humans. *Clinical and Experimental Immunology, 167*, 261−268.

Park, Y. J., & Luger, K. (2008). Histone chaperones in nucleosome eviction and histone exchange. *Current Opinion in Structural Biology, 18*, 282−289.

Parker, H., Dragunow, M., Hampton, M. B., Kettle, A. J., & Winterbourn, C. C. (2012). Requirements for NADPH oxidase and myeloperoxidase in neutrophil extracellular trap formation differ depending on the stimulus. *Journal of Leukocyte Biology, 92*, 841−849.

Patel, S., Kumar, S., & Jyoti, A. (2010). 'Nitric oxide donors release extracellular traps from human neutrophils by augmenting free radical generation. *Nitric Oxide, 22*(3), 226−234.

Pedersen, F., Marwitz, S., Holz, O., Kirsten, A., Bahmer, T., & Waschki, B. (2015). Neutrophil extracellular trap formation and extracellular DNA in sputum of stable COPD patients. *Respiratory Medicine, 109*, 1360−1362. Available from https://doi.org/10.1016/j.rmed.2015.08.008.

Perdomo, J. J., Gounon, P., & Sansonetti, P. J. (1994). Polymorphonuclear leukocyte transmigration promotes invasion of colonic epithelial monolayer by *Shigella flexneri*. *Journal of Clinical Investigation, 93*, 633−643. Available from https://doi.org/10.1172/JCI117011.

Persson, Y. A., Blomgran-Julinder, R., Rahman, S., Zheng, L., & Stendahl, O. (2008). *Mycobacterium tuberculosis*-induced apoptotic neutrophils trigger a proinflammatory response in macrophages through release of heat shock protein 72, acting in synergy with the bacteria. *Microbes and Infection, 10*, 233−240. Available from https://doi.org/10.1016/j.micinf.2007.11.007.

Phalipon, A., & Sansonetti, P. J. (2007). Shigellas ways of manipulating the host intestinal innate and adaptive immune system: A tool box for survival? *Immunology and Cell Biology, 85*, 119−129. Available from https://doi.org/10.1038/sj.icb7100025.

Price, M. O., Atkinson, S. J., & Knaus, U. G. (2002). Rac activation induces NADPH oxidase activity in transgenic COSphox cells, and the level of superoxide production is exchange factor-dependent. *The Journal of biological chemistry, 277*, 19220−19228.

Qiu, S. L., Zhang, H., Tang, Q. Y., Bai, J., He, Z. Y., Zhang, J. Q., ... Zhong, X. N. (2017). Neutrophil extracellular traps induced by cigarette smoke activate plasmacytoid dendritic cells. *Thorax, 72*, 1084−1093.

Ramos-Kichik, V., Mondragon-Flores, R., Mondragon-Castelan, M., GonzalezPozos, S., Muniz-Hernandez, S., & Rojas-Espinosa, O. (2009). Neutrophil extracellular traps are induced by *Mycobacterium tuberculosis*. *Tuberculosis, 89*, 29−37. Available from https://doi.org/10.1016/j.tube.2008.09.00.

Reidl, J., & Klose, K. E. (2002). *Vibrio cholerae* and cholera: Out of the water and into the host. *FEMS Microbiological Reviews, 26*, 125−139. Available from https://doi.org/10.1111/j.1574-6976.2002.tb00605.

Rocha, J. D., Nascimento, M. T., Decote-Ricardo, D., Corte-Real, S., Morrot, A., & Heise, N. (2015). Capsular polysaccharides from *Cryptococcus neoformans* modulate production of neutrophil extracellular traps (NETs) by human neutrophils. *Scientific Reports, 5*, 8008. Available from https://doi.org/10.1038/srep08008.

Rodriguez-Espinosa, O., Rojas-Espinosa, O., Moreno-Altamirano, M. M., LopezVillegas, E. O., & Sanchez-Garcia, F. J. (2015). Metabolic requirements for neutrophil extracellular traps formation. *Immunology, 145*, 213−224. Available from https://doi.org/10.1111/imm.1243.

Seeley, E. J., Matthay, M. A., & Wolters, P. J. (2012). Inflection points in sepsis biology: From local defense to systemic organ injury. *American Journal of Physiology Lung Cellular and Molecular Physiology, 303*, L355−L363. Available from https://doi.org/10.1152/ajplung.00069.2012.

Segal, B. H., & Romani, L. R. (2009). Invasive aspergillosis in chronic granulomatous disease. *Medical Mycology, 47*, S282−S290. Available from https://doi.org/10.1080/13693780902736620.

Seper, A., Hosseinzadeh, A., Gorkiewicz, G., Lichtenegger, S., Roier, S., & Leitner, D. R. (2013). *Vibrio cholerae* evades neutrophil extracellular traps by the activity of two extracellular nucleases. *PLoS Pathogen, 9*, e1003614. Available from https://doi.org/10.1371/journal.ppat.1003614.

Sollberger, G., Amulic, B., & Zychlinsky, A. (2016). Neutrophil extracellular trap formation is independent of de novo gene expression. *PLoS One, 11*, e0157454.

Sorg, J. A., & Sonenshein, A. L. (2010). Inhibiting the initiation of Clostridium difficile spore germination using analogs of chenodeoxycholic acid, a bile acid. *Journal of Bacteriology, 192*, 4983−4990. Available from https://doi.org/10.1128/JB.00610-10.

Sousa-Rocha, D., Thomaz-Tobias, M., Diniz, L. F., Souza, P. S., Pinge-Filho, P., & Toledo, K. A. (2015). *Trypanosoma cruzi* and its soluble antigens induce NET release by stimulating toll-like receptors. *PLoS One, 10*, e0139569.

Spinner, J. L., Seo, K. S., OLoughlin, J. L., Cundiff, J. A., Minnich, S. A., & Bohach, G. A. (2010). Neutrophils are resistant to Yersinia YopJ/P-induced apoptosis and are protected from ROS-mediated cell death by the type III secretion system. *PLoS One, 5*, e9279. Available from https://doi.org/10.1371/journal.pone.0009279.

Steinberg, B. E., & Grinstein, S. (2007). Unconventional roles of the NADPH oxidase: Signaling, ion homeostasis, and cell death. *Science STKE, 379*, pe11.

Talbert, P. B., & Henikoff, S. (2010). Histone variants—ancient wrap artists of the epigenome. *Nature Review of Molecular Cell Biology, 11*, 264−275.

Tammavongsa, V., Missiakas, D. M., & Schneewind, O. (2014). *Staphylococcus aureus* degrades neutrophil extracellular traps to promote immune cell death. *Science, 342*, 863−866. Available from https://doi.org/10.1126/science.1242255.

Tanaka, K., Koike, Y., Shimura, T., Okigami, M., Ide, S., & Toiyama, Y. (2014). In vivo characterization of neutrophil extracellular traps in various organs of a murine sepsis model. *PLoS One, 9*, e111888. Available from https://doi.org/10.1371/journal.pone.0111888.

Tobias, A. F., Ulrike, A., Christian, G., Robert, H., Ilka, S., & Volker, W. (2007). Novel cell death program leads to neutrophil extracellular traps. *Journal of Cell Biology, 176*(2), 231−241. Available from https://doi.org/10.1083/jcb.200606027.

Tripathi, S., Verma, A., Kim, E. J., White, M. R., & Hartshorn, K. L. (2014). LL-37 modulates human neutrophil responses to influenza A virus. *Journal of Leukocyte Biology, 96*, 931−938. Available from https://doi.org/10.1189/jlb.4A1113-604RR.

Troeger, A., & Williams, D. A. (2013). Hematopoietic-specific Rho GTPases Rac2 and RhoH and human blood disorders. *Experimental Cell Research, 319*, 2375−2383.

Urban, C. F. (2009). Neutrophil extracellular traps contain Calprotectin, a cytosolic protein complex involved in host defense against *Candida albicans*. *PLoS Pathogens, 5*, e1000639.

Urban, C. F., Ermert, D., Schmid, M., Abu-Abed, U., Goosmann, C., Nacken, W., ... Zychlinsky, A. (2009). Neutrophil extracellular traps contain calprotectin, a cytosolic protein complex involved in host defense against *Candida albicans*. *PLoS Pathogens, 5*, e1000639.

Van Dervort, A. L., Yan, L., Madara, P. J., Cobb, J. P., & Wesley, R. A. (1994). Nitric oxide regulates endotoxin-induced TNF-alpha production by human neutrophils. *Journal of Immunology, 152*, 4102−4109.

von Kökritz-Blickwede, M., Goldmann, O., Tulin, P., Heinemann, K., NorrbyTeglund, A., & Rohde, M. (2008). Phagocytosis-independent antimicrobial activity of mast cells by means of extracellular trap formation. *Blood, 111*(6), 3070−3080. Available from https://doi.org/10.1182/blood-2007-07-104018.

Vorobjeva, N. V. (2013). NADPH oxidase of neutrophils and diseases associated with its dysfunction. *Immunologiya, 34*, 232238.

Waisberg, M., Molina-Cruz, A., Mizurini, D. M., Gera, N., Sousa, B. C., & Ma, D. (2014). *Plasmodium falciparum* infection induces expression of a mosquito salivary protein (Agaphelin) that targets neutrophil function and inhibits thrombosis without impairing hemostasis. *PLoS Pathogens, 10*, e1004338. Available from https://doi.org/10.1371/journal.ppat.100433.

Wang, Y., Li, M., Stadler, S., Correll, S., Li, P., Wang, D., . . . Coonrod, S. A. (2009). Histone hypercitrullination mediates chromatin decondensation and neutrophil extracellular trap formation. *Journal of Cell Biology, 184*, 205−213.

Wartha, F., Beiter, K., Albiger, B., Fernebro, J., Zychlinsky, A., & Normark, S. (2007). Capsule and D-alanylated lipoteichoic acids protect *Streptococcus pneumoniae* against neutrophil extracellular traps. *Cellular Microbiology, 9*(5), 1162−1171. Available from https://doi.org/10.1111/j.1462-5822.2006.00857.x.

Wildhagen, K. C., Garcia de Frutos, P., Reutelingsperger, C. P., Schrijver, R., Areste, C., Ortega-Gomez, A., . . . Nicolaes, G. A. (2014). Nonanticoagulant heparin prevents histone-mediated cytotoxicity in vitro and improves survival in sepsis. *Blood, 123*, 1098−1101.

Wu, F., Tyml, K., & Wilson, J. X. (2008). iNOS expression requires NADPH oxidase-dependent redox signaling in microvascular endothelial cells. *Journal of Cellular Physiology, 217*, 207−214.

Xu, J., Zhang, X., Pelayo, R., Monestier, M., Ammollo, C. T., Semeraro, F., . . . Esmon, C. T. (2009). Extracellular histones are major mediators of death in sepsis. *Nature Medicine, 15*, 1318−1321.

Yang, H., & Biermann, M. H. (2016). New insights into neutrophil extracellular traps: Mechanisms of formation and role in inflammation. *Frontiers in Immunology, 7*, 1−8. Available from https://doi.org/10.3389/fimmu.2016.00302.

Young, R. L., Malcolm, K. C., Kret, J. E., Caceres, S. M., Poch, K. R., & Nichols, D. P. (2011). Neutrophil extracellular trap (NET)-mediated killing of *Pseudomonas aeruginosa*: Evidence of acquired resistance within the CF airway, independent of CFTR. *PLoS One, 6*, e23637. Available from https://doi.org/10.1371/journal.pone.0023637.

Zhu, L., Kuang, Z., Wilson, B. A., & Lau, G. W. (2013). Competence-independent activity of pneumococcal EndA [corrected] mediates degradation of extracellular DNA and nets and is important for virulence. *PLoS One, 8*, e70363. Available from https://doi.org/10.1371/journal.pone.0070363.

Zigra, P. I., Maipa, V. E., & Alamanos, Y. P. (2007). Probiotics and remission of ulcerative colitis: A systematic review. *Netherlands Journal of Medicine, 65*, 411−418.

Chapter 2

NETosis: mechanisms and antimicrobial strategies

The process of extracellular trap formation during NETosis involves an intricate course with several successive steps including: reactive oxygen species (ROS) formation followed by transport of neutrophil elastase (NE), and subsequently, of myeloperoxidase (MPO) from the granules to the nucleus; unwinding of DNA from nucleosomes caused by histone modifications, and, finally disruption of cytoplasmic membrane and release of chromatin (Fig. 2.1). Designing relevant experimental procedures to study NETosis mechanisms is challenging, which is further complicated by the use of pharmacologic inducers of NETosis. Despite these impediments, reasonable advances in the understanding of the mechanisms of NETosis have been made.

NETosis inducing stimuli can be roughly categorized into pathogen associated triggers, or inflammatory or endogenous triggers. Pathogen associated physiological stimuli include viruses, bacteria, protozoa, and fungi. ROS mediated NETosis can be induced by substances such as antibodies (Kessenbrock, Krumbholz, & Schönermarck, 2009) and antigen−antibody complexes (Garcia Romo et al., 2011; Lande et al., 2011) hydrogen peroxide (Fuchs et al., 2007); constituents from microbes such as, lipopolysaccharide (LPS) (Lim, Kuiper, Katchky, Goldberg, & Glogauer, 2011; Neeli, Dwivedi, Khan, & Radic, 2009), the lipophosphoglycans present in *Leishmania amazonensis* (Guimaraes Costa et al., 2009) and M1 protein in *Streptococcus pyogenes* (Oehmcke, Morgelin, & Herwald, 2009). Extracellular traps can also be induced by Toll-like receptor (TLR4) activated platelets (Clark et al., 2007). A diverse array of signaling receptors on neutrophils can induce NETosis, such as binding via TLRs, Fc receptors, or complement receptors have been implicated in the neutrophil extracellular trap (NET) induction (Farquharson, Butcher, & Culshaw, 2012; Steinberg & Grinstein, 2007; Vorobjeva, 2013). Cytokine receptors may also be associated with NETosis signaling as like IL-8, TNF, and IFN-γ have shown to trigger NETosis (Neeli et al., 2009; Papayannopoulos, Metzler, Hakkim, & Zychlinsky, 2010; Steinberg & Grinstein, 2007). Further studies are warranted to address the interaction or cross talk between different categories of neutrophil receptors involved in the induction of NETosis

NETosis. DOI: https://doi.org/10.1016/B978-0-12-816147-0.00002-2

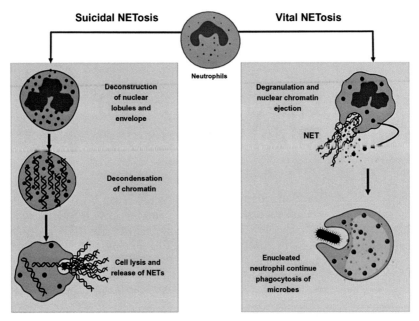

FIGURE 2.1 NET formation pathways: there are two routes of NET formation. First route starts with delobulation of the nucleus and nuclear envelope disassembly, followed by loss of cellular polarization, decondensation of chromatin, and rupture of plasma membrane. Second route employs secreted expulsion of nuclear chromatin along with granular protein release through degranulation, which takes place without cell lysis. These components integrate extracellularly leaving anucleated cytoplasts behind with retained ability of ingesting microorganisms.

Role of DNA and histones in neutrophil extracellular trap release

DNA in NETosis

A prerequisite for NET formation is the deployment of nuclear material from the nucleus to the environment. Many eukaryotic cells routinely disintegrate their nuclear envelope, even without NADPH oxidase, to facilitate DNA division. Molecular mechanisms of how neutrophils release DNA from the nucleus may be obtained by evaluating how other cells undergo nuclear division. An outer and inner lipid membrane serves as the constituents of the nuclear envelope along with aqueous pore complexes structurally clutched conjointly by intermediate protein filaments called lamina, which can be shredded open by microtubules. The nuclear envelop may break down rapidly as evident from biphasic mechanisms observed in oocytes wherein partial disassembly of the pore complex takes place in about 10 minutes. Following this complete permeabilization takes place within 35 seconds and finally, complete dissociation of the lamina takes place in additional 10 minutes

(Lénárt et al., 2003) and requires microtubules (Beaudouin, Gerlich, Daigle, Eils, & Ellenberg, 2002). However, the evidence of these mechanisms also occurring in neutrophils is currently unclear just as their requirement for release of DNA into the cytoplasm erstwhile NET release. This suggests that neutrophils are likely to engage distinctive mechanisms of nuclear envelope break down. An example of this, the relocation of elastase to the nucleus as a precondition for NET release, yet most of the elastase is, limited to the neutrophil.

Microbicidal activity of DNA in neutrophil extracellular traps

There have been reports of DNA possessing rapid bactericidal activity due to its capacity to sequester surface bound cations, disrupt membrane integrity, and lyse bacterial cells. However, direct contact and the phosphodiester backbone are needed for the cation chelating, antimicrobial property of DNA. Treatment of NETs with surplus cations or phosphatase enzyme neutralizes the antimicrobial activity of NETs, but maintains NET structure, including the localization and function of NET-bound proteins (Halverson, Wilton, Poon, Petri, & Lewenza, 2015).

Major proteins involved in NETosis

The primary protein constituents of NETs are histones, trailed by granular enzymes and peptides including NE, MPO, cathepsin G, leukocyte proteinase 3 (PR3), lactoferrin, gelatinase, lysozyme C, calprotectin, neutrophil defensins, and cathelicidins (Urban et al., 2009). The term NET was used to refer to the collection of these along with released chromatin structures and this unusual cell death route was named NETosis consequently (Steinberg & Grinstein, 2007). A plethora of NETosis inducers have been described, including bacteria or bacterial components (Brinkmann et al., 2004), protozoa (Aulik, Hellenbrand, Klos, & Czuprynski, 2010; Sousa-Rocha et al., 2015), fungi (Grinstein, 2007), viruses (Saitoh et al., 2012), complement-derived peptides (Yousefi, Mihalache, Kozlowski, Schmid, & Simon, 2009), activated platelets (Saitoh et al., 2012), autoantibodies (Kessenbrock et al., 2009), IL-8 (Brinkmann et al., 2004), urate crystals (Mitroulis et al., 2011), hydrogen peroxide (Fuchs et al., 2007), cigarette smoke (Qiu et al., 2017), and ionophores (Parker, Dragunow, Hampton, Kettle, & Winterbourn, 2012).

NADPH-mediated NETs also help avert infections as patients with chronic granulomatous disease (CGD) (a primary immunodeficiency disease that causes respiratory burst in phagocytic leukocytes) endure repeated infections due to an inoperative NADPH oxidase complex. Utilizing gene therapy to restore its function rebuilds the ability to form NETs and to overcome fungal lung infections (Bianchi et al., 2009). During NETosis NE is assembled together with MPO and is carried to the nucleus wherein it processes core histones (Metzler, Goosmann, Lubojemska, Zychlinsky, & Papayannopoulos, 2014; Papayannopoulos et al., 2010). This causes an elevation in the intracellular calcium levels that activates peptidyl arginine deiminase 4 (PAD4), which converts arginine in histones to citrulline, leading to a decline in the positive charge of these proteins (Neeli et al., 2009; Neeli, Khan, & Radic, 2008; Wang et al., 2009). Collectively, these molecular events decrease the compaction of chromatin. Subsequently, after about 2 hour, Phorbol-12-myristate-13-acetate (PMA)-induced neutrophils lose heterochromatic areas of the nucleus as well as the characteristic nuclear lobuli. As a consequence nuclei round up and expand. The nuclear envelope collapses into vesicles, granules, and mitochondria break down. Cytoplasm and karyoplasm intermix and finally the cell membrane bursts and discharges the cellular content, which unfolds in the extracellular space to form NETs (Fuchs et al., 2007).

Histones in neutrophil extracellular trap

First defined by Albrecht Kossel in 1884, histones are histidine-rich peptones originating from the nuclear component of avian red blood cells. Histones are nuclear chaperone proteins that are greatly conserved across all eukaryotes (Talbert & Henikoff, 2010), and interacts with nucleic acids due to the highly positive charge (Park & Luger, 2008) conferred by lysine and arginine residues. About 147 base pairs of DNA are wrapped around each nucleosome in 1.7 turns by the histone protein octamer composed of core histones (H2A, H2B, H3, and H4), further compacted by linker histones (H1 and/or H5) (Luger, Mader, Richmond, Sargent, & Richmond, 2011). This forms the compact chromatin structure of DNA. The release of DNA in NETosis requires relaxation of the tightly bound DNA from the histones.

Various posttranslational modifications of histones that aid in the process of NETosis have been recognized, including acetylation, methylation, phosphorylation, sumoylation, ADP ribosylation, ubiquitylion, deimination, and proline isomerization (Kouzarides, 2007). In a typical cell function this modifies the makeup of the histone DNA interface and permit transcription to occur. Decondensation of chromatin and release of genomic DNA due to controlled histone degradation has been described in NETs (Brinkmann et al., 2004; Papayannopoulos et al., 2010). These mesh-work like structures assists in intravascular thrombosis (Fuchs, Brill, & Duerschmied, 2010), limit spread of microorganisms, encourage cancer metastasis (Cools-Lartigue, Spicer, & McDonald, 2013), and cause direct injury to adjacent cells (Allam, Kumar, Darisipudi, & Anders, 2014).

Histones as damage-associated molecular patterns

Among the earliest and better described ways in which histones aggravate cellular injury is in their role as alarmins or damage-associated molecular patterns (DAMPS). Histones are one of the initially recognized and well-described alarmins or DAMPS that aggravates cellular injury. Necrotic cells eject histones inactively (or actively by other modes of cell death including NETosis) act on nearby cells and circulating immune cells via pattern recognition receptors to result in distinctive biological activity. These observations are difficult to interpret in vivo systems as histones are coreleased with nuclear DNA and other nuclear DAMPs such as HMGB1 (high mobility group box protein 1), each with their individual activities.

The cytotoxicity of histones is well expressed as antihistone antibodies have been reported to prevent pathogenesis in various disease models (Wildhagen et al., 2014; Xu et al., 2009). Huge amounts of histones are released by NETs into tissues where they not only target microbes but also cause tissue damage. Certainly this emphasizes that the antimicrobial function of NETs might be, at least partially, due to histones and they are likely to impact the pathogenic effect of NETs.

Of the various posttranslational histone modifications that mediate gene expression and chromatin structure (reviewed by Bannister & Kouzarides, 2011), one modification previously stated in NETosis is "clipping" by serine proteases which might enable chromatin decondensation and subsequent DNA release. Histones are also found to be citrullinated in NETs (Dwivedi et al., 2014) where there is a conversion of arginine to citrulline (a nonencoded amino acid) by peptidylarginine deiminases (PADs). PAD4 is involved in histone citrullination during NETosis in vitro, and chemical or genetic removal of PAD4 lessens NET formation (Knight et al., 2013; Knight et al., 2015; Lewis et al., 2015; Li, Li, Lindberg, Kennett, Xiong, & Wang, 2010). However, the requirement of PAD4 for NETosis is still questionable.

Reactive oxygen species as key factor in NETosis

Evidence of ROS as a key player in classical suicidal NETosis pathway has surfaced from mainly two distinct observations: firstly, patients with CGD show reduced NET forming ability from their neutrophils as these neutrophils are not capable of mediating the oxidative burst. However, this is distinct from the NETosis ablation caused by defective phagocytic oxidase (PHOX) complex wherein treatment with H_2O_2 rescues the production of NETs, downstream of PHOX complex in CGD patients (Tobias et al., 2007). Second, NETosis inhibition also takes place in presence of ROS scavengers such as N-acetylcysteine or trolox (Tobias et al., 2007). However, the role of ROS in disassembling of the nuclear envelope or mixing of components of NETs is still unclear. Some of the studies indicate that ROS is involved in stimulating morphological changes noticed during NETosis (Kaplan & Marko, 2012). ROS may otherwise inactivate caspases, thus impeding apoptosis and supporting autophagy, leading to the dissolution of cellular membranes (Remijsen, Berghe, & Wirawan, 2011). These two pathways are independent under varied experimental conditions and not simply mutually exclusive. Growing number of evidences support the fact that NADPH oxidase independent NETosis is induced by certain stimuli (Parker et al., 2012) described later in the chapter.

ROS formation in neutrophils takes place during the purported "respiratory burst" which involves the NADPH oxidase complex (Vorobjeva, 2013). Assembly of this multicomponent enzyme complex takes place during activation in membranes of specific granules, on the cytoplasmic membrane of neutrophils and is primarily involved in the transfer of electrons from NADPH localized in the cytoplasm through the membrane to molecular oxygen. Then reduction of one electron in oxygen takes place, forming superoxide anion radical (O_2^-) Thereafter, it undergoes redox transformation, concomitantly or with the association of superoxide dismutase (SOD) with hydrogen peroxide (H_2O_2) as by-product. Further transformation of these primary ROS [(O_2^-) and $H_2O_2^-$] ensuing the production of more active metabolites, for example, hydroxyl radical (OH·) and hypochlorous acid (HOCl) takes place. One of the strongest microbicidal effect is produced by HOCl, and is formed with the involvement of MPO, the enzyme of azurophilic granules.

MPO forms an important part of the "azurosome," a protein complex, residing in azurophilic granules and containing eight proteins, which includes three highly homologous serine proteases NE, cathepsin G, and azurocidin. These small proteases, although lacking nuclear localization signals, can passively diffuse into the nucleus. This takes place as hydrogen peroxide triggers azurosome dissociation causing leakage of these serine proteases into the cytoplasm from where they are proposed to migrate to the nucleus (Metzler et al., 2014). Clipping of histones in the nucleus then takes place mediated by these serine proteases, enabling chromatin relaxation.

Cell-cycle kinases in reactive oxygen species−dependent NETosis

One of the surprising factors of NADPH oxidase−dependent NETosis is the requirement of activation of cyclin-dependent kinases (CDKs) in terminally differentiated neutrophils to draw out of its resting G_0 stage and enter into the cell cycle (Amulic et al., 2017). The markers exclusive for NETosis undergoing neutrophils are the proliferative markers Ki-67, and CDK6 is involved in the phosphorylation of its cell cycle substrate, retinoblastoma protein, during NET formation. Dependably, CDK6-deficient mice are more prone to infection. The events of S-phase comprising synthesis of DNA and transcription of histone genes, do not take place during NETosis. Unexpectedly the events of M-phase like lamin phosphorylation and centrosome separation are involved in NET formation. This emphasizes the use of cellular machinery in disassembly of the nuclear membrane by neutrophils.

Reactive oxygen species–independent NETosis

NETosis can also take place in a NADPH oxidase/ROS-independent manner without the need for NE and identified by citrullinated histone H3. First observed in calcium ionophore A23187, a NET inducer produced through the growth of *Streptomyces chartreusensis* and another inducer, potassium ionophore nigericin, derived from the bacteria *Streptomyces hygroscopicus*, do not require NADPH oxidase or MPO activity (Kenny et al., 2017; Neeli & Radic, 2013). Although two of the pathways for NETosis are supported by various experimental data; however, the mechanisms involved in NET release is still not well understood. The NETosis mediators present in neutrophils do not require de novo gene expression and are neither the NADPH oxidase–dependent nor NADPH oxidase–independent (Kenny et al., 2017; Sollberger, Amulic, & Zychlinsky, 2016). Notably similar to the canonical form the alternative NETosis is distinct from necroptosis (Kenny et al., 2017), apoptosis (Remijsen et al., 2011), and other forms of cell death. Particularly, NET formation can depend on mitochondrial (Lood et al., 2016) or pathogen (Kenny et al., 2017) derived ROS through a pathway that remains to be described in detail.

Recently the role of Gasdermin-D (GSDMD), a pore-forming protein and executor of pyroptosis, is demonstrated to play a vital role in NET formation (Sollberger et al., 2018). In neutrophils, serine proteases, like NE, cleaves GSDMD and permits the discharge of granular proteins that are required for NETosis progression in a feed-forward loop. GSDMD-dependent NETosis can also take place by activation of noncanonical inflammasomes in neutrophils as reported by Chen et al. (2018). These two studies together demonstrate how GSDMD acts as an important executioner in response to different stimuli that activate diverse proteases to cleave GSDMD and induce NETosis. Nonclassical or vital NETosis requires intracellular LPS that promote inflammasome assembly and caspase cleavage of GSDMD, whereas classical NETosis requires ROS activating serine proteases that also cleave GSDMD. This establishes GSDMD as a hub of proinflammatory cell death.

Signaling pathways involved in NETosis

The signaling pathways involved in NETosis are diverse (Fig. 2.2) as these involve various immune cell receptors that can be triggered by signals induced by microorganisms and endogenous stimuli such as DAMPs and immune complexes.

Rac2 signaling pathway

Rac is a subfamily of Rho GTPases (guanosine triphosphatases), which coordinate cellular response to extracellular signals with the help of highly conserved low molecular weight proteins that act as molecular switches

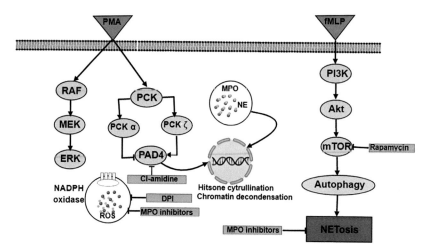

FIGURE 2.2   Molecular mechanisms regulating NETosis. PMA is one of the well-known factors inducing suicidal NETosis. Under its influence the Raf−MEK−ERK pathway and protein kinase C are activated, resulting in the stimulation of the NADPH oxidase complex and ROS formation. PAD4 is also activated, contributing to histone citrullination. MPO and NE released from azurophilic granules move to the cell nucleus, where they initiate further decondensation of nuclear chromatin, and then, bind with the proteins originating from granules and the cytoplasm. The structure thus formed at the time of cellular membrane disruption is released into the extracellular space, which results in cell death. It has been observed that the process of ROS transformation by MPO inside the neutrophil granules plays an important role in the NETs generation. This is indicated by the fact that the phenomenon can be inhibited by the use of MPO inhibitors. Rapamycin used in this study inhibits mTOR kinase, contributing to an increase in the autophagic activity, thus accelerating the NETs release by fMLP-stimulated neutrophils. *MEK*, MAPK/ERK kinase; *mTOR*, mechanistic target of rapamycin; *PI3K*, phosphoinositide 3-kinase; *PKC*, protein kinase C; *RIPK1*, receptor-interacting serine/threonine-protein kinase 1; *TLR*, Toll-like receptor; *MPO*, myeloperoxidase; *fMLP*, N-Formylmethionine-leucyl-phenylalanine; *DPI*, diphenyleneiodonium-inhibitor of ROS.

(Troeger & Williams, 2013). Rac proteins are categorized into three highly homologous proteins based on their expression levels—Rac1, Rac2, and Rac3, which play a central role in regulating response to inflammatory signals mediated by neutrophils, including chemotaxis, actin cytoskeleton remodeling, and production of superoxide by NADPH oxidase (Dinauer, 2003). Rac after being activated [guanosine triphosphate (GTP) bound] plays two roles in NADPH activation which include triggering oxidase complex assembly and functioning as an enzyme subunit (Babior, 1999; Price, Atkinson, & Knaus, 2002). Rho GTPases are primarily activated by the vav family of guanine nucleotide exchange factors (GEFs) by catalyzing the exchange of guanosine diphosphate for GTP. The downstream effectors of Rac proteins are p21-activated kinases (Paks). Pak alters conformation, translocate to the plasma membrane, combines with the catalytic part of the NADPH complex and phosphorylates p47 PHOX resulting in a complex regulatory component necessary for ROS production (Martyn, Kim, & Quinn, 2005). Studies on Rac2 signaling pathway have shed some light on NETosis signals. During this pathway, phosphorylation of gp91phox by protein kinase C (PKC) permits the assembly of cytosolic and membrane-bound subunits of NADPH oxidase into a functional complex that produces ROS and, specifically, superoxide ions (Raad et al., 2009). While neutrophils lacking Rac1 release similar quantities of NET chromatin as wild-type neutrophils when induced with PMA or LPS, Rac2-deficient cells fail to develop a functional enzyme complex and have compromised NET formation (Lim et al., 2011). Furthermore, NET release also requires conversion of superoxide to hydrogen peroxide and to perchloric acid. However, superoxide itself is dispensable, as neutrophils in patients with CGD showed rescue of the NETosis pathway upon addition of exogenous peroxide.

Raf/MEK/ERK signaling pathway

Ras/Raf/MEK/ERK signaling cascade is used by growth factors and mitogens to transmit signals from their receptors by coupling signals from cell surface receptors to transcription factors, regulating gene expression, and preventing apoptosis. Ras proteins belong to the class of small GTPases that induce translocation of Raf, a serine/threonine-specific protein kinase, to the cell membrane. Raf promotes MEK1/2 (MAPK/ERK kinase), which is a dual specificity protein kinase, that activates ERK1/2. This activated ERK1/2 phosphorylates several substrates and regulates different transcription factors, leading to different gene expressions. By activating NADPH oxidase and upregulating antiapoptotic proteins, Raf−MEK−ERK pathway is involved in NET formation. MEK/ERK signaling is triggered by a variety of receptors that include P-selectin glycoprotein ligand 1 (PSGL1), HMGB-receptor for advanced glycation end products (RAGE), Complement receptor 3 (CR3), TLR2/4, Siglec-14, and FcγR. The molecules implicated in signal transduction from the receptors to NADPH oxidase were discovered by rigorous inhibition analysis carried out in the laboratory of Zychlinsky (Kenny et al., 2017). PMA, the most effective and frequently used NETosis activator, is the immediate stimulator of PKC. PMA induced NETosis by PMA is accompanied by the induction of the Raf/MEK/ERK signaling pathway (Kenny et al., 2017), as well as the Rac2 (a small GTPase of the Rho family)-mediated pathway (Raad et al., 2009).

PI3K/AKT/mTOR pathway

The PI3K/AKT/mTOR pathway is a cell cycle regulating pathway which transduces signals intracellularly. Therefore it promotes metabolism, proliferation, cell survival, growth, and angiogenesis in response to extracellular signals. Phosphatidylinositol 3-kinase (PI3K) is capable of phosphorylating the $3'$ position hydroxyl group of the inositol ring of phosphatidylinositol. PI3K consists of two domains: a catalytic domain P110 and a regulatory domain P85. The activation of PI3K typically occurs as a result of direct stimulation via the regulatory subunit bound to the activated receptor or indirectly activated via adapter molecules such as the insulin receptor substrate proteins. PI3K can also be activated by a GTP-binding RAS protein. In PI3K-AKT pathway the $3'$ position phosphate group of PIP3 can bind to both PDK1 and AKT protein and recruiting AKT protein at the plasma membrane, allowing PDK1 to access and phosphorylate T308 in the "activation loop," leading to partial PKB/Akt activation. Then the phosphorylation of Akt at S473 in the carboxy-terminal hydrophobic motif, either by mTORC2 or by DNA-PK, stimulates full Akt activity. Akt also named as protein kinase B, is a serine/threonine-specific protein kinase, that plays a key role in multiple cellular processes. Once activated, Akt regulates the function via phosphorylation activation or suppression of a broad array of proteins involved in cell growth, proliferation, motility, adhesion, neovascularization, and death.

PI3K is also required for NETosis which has also been implicated for a role in autophagy, which also depends on this enzyme (Remijsen et al., 2011). Similar to this, promyelocytes lacking autophagy-associated protein, ATG7, exhibited a small decrease in NET release (Ma et al., 2016). By analogy a requirement for mechanistic target of rapamycin (mTOR), which suppresses autophagy has also been implicated in NETosis (McInturff et al., 2012). Nonetheless, LC3B$^+$ vacuoles that resemble autophagosomes have been observed in neutrophils undergoing NETosis (Remijsen et al., 2011; Tang et al., 2015; Ma et al., 2016). Finally, ROS are known to induce autophagy (Bhattacharya et al., 2015; Filomeni, De Zio, & Cecconi, 2015), which in turn is required to sustain the ROS burst and might also help to tolerate ROS-induced stress.

Other kinases involved in neutrophil extracellular trap signaling

During NETosis, permeabilization of plasma membrane occurs in an organized step-wise manner and not as a result of expanding chromatin that causes physical disruption of the plasma membrane (Metzler et al., 2014). This observation aligns with the supposed involvement of NETosis and programmed cell death. In accordance with this observation, inducers of NET, such as monosodium urate (MSU) crystals, stimulate necroptosis, and neutrophils lacking receptor-interacting serine/threonine-protein kinase 1 (RIPK1) and RIPK3, two kinases involved in necroptosis, fail to form NETs without altering their ROS burst, which indicates that these enzymes act downstream or in parallel with the ROS pathway (Desai et al., 2016). However, the role of these kinases in NETosis has been challenged by others (Amini et al., 2016), and more evidences are required to confirm their role and mode of action.

Antimicrobial strategies of neutrophil extracellular traps

A significantly copious amount of microbes seemingly induce formation of NETs (Table 2.1). These instigator NET-inducing molecules include components of the bacterial cell surface molecules like LPS, lipoteichoic acid, and their breakdown products. Of the potential NET-inducing bacteria and fungi, the ones that are apparent are, *Staphylococcus aureus*, *Streptococcus* sp., *Haemophilus influenzae*, *Klebsiella pneumonia*, *Listeria monocytogenes*, *Mycobacterium tuberculosis*, *Shigella flexneri*, *Aspergillus nidulans*, *Aspergillus fumigatus*, and *Candida albicans* (Yang & Biermann, 2016). In addition, pathogens, such as *Yersinia* (Brinkmann et al., 2004) and members of the oral microbiome, including *Porphyromonas gingivalis* also induce NET formation (Delbosc et al., 2011). Being web-like traps of cells that splurt out during an infection, NETs can restrain and kill a broad range of microbes, including bacteria, fungi, and protozoa (Brinkmann et al., 2004; Papayannopoulos et al., 2010;

TABLE 2.1 Different inducers employ different signaling pathways in NETosis.

Inducing agent		Receptors involved in activation	Intermediate proteins involved in signal transduction	Pathway
Microbes	Bacteria	Siglec-14, TLR4	PAD4, NOX2, MPO, NE	ND
	Viruses	TLR7, TLR8	ND	ND
	Fungi	CR3, Dectin 2	MPO, NOX2, NE	ND
	Parasites	TLR2, TLR4	ND	NOX2 independent
Compounds or complexes	Crystals	ND	MPO, RIPK1, RIPK3, NOX2, NE	PAD4 independent
	PMA	NA	RIPK1, RIPK3, MEK, ERK, NOX2, AKT, PI3K, mTOR, ATG7, MPO, NE, DEK	PAD4 independent
	Ionomycin	ND	mitoROS, NE, PAD4, SK3, PKC7,	ERK, NOX2 independent
	LPS and/or platelets	TLR2, TLR4, PSGL1, RAGE	HMGB1, NE	NOX2 independent
	Immune complexes	FcγRIIIb	mitoROS	NOX2 independent

Pilsczek et al., 2010; Urban, Reichard, Brinkmann, & Zychlinsky, 2006; von Kökritz-Blickwede et al., 2008), and thus avert the spreading of microbial pathogens (Juneau, Pang, Weimer, Armbruster, & Swords, 2011). However, the killing capabilities are debatable as some experiments revealed that NETs upon treatment with DNases release bound *S. aureus* and *C. albicans* blastospores which imply that NETs might be just trapping structures and are not antimicrobials.

According to data, neutrophils selectively released NETs in response to large pathogens, like filamentous *C. albicans* (Branzk et al., 2014). Interestingly, yeast form of *C. albicans* or single bacteria could not induce NETosis. Phagocytosis mediated by dectin-1 functioned as a microbial size sensor and prevented release of NET by downregulating translocation of NE to the nucleus. In addition to directly killing microbes, NETs also act by inactivating microbial "virulence factors" that alter host cell functions. The virulence factors of *S. flexneri*, *Salmonella typhimurium*, and *Yersinia enterocolitica* are specifically cleaved by NET-associated NE (Brinkmann et al., 2004). Other classes of microbes are destroyed by the serine proteases cathepsin G and PR3 that destroy virulence factors of these classes of microbes (Averhoff, Kolbe, Zychlinsky, & Weinrauch, 2008). Several microbe inhibiting proteins are present in NETs such as enzymes, antimicrobial peptides (AMPs), calgranulin, and histones. The combined action of several components is being enhanced by microbicidal activity of NETs resulting from the high local concentrations of mediators on the NETs' surfaces (Pilsczek et al., 2010).

The bactericidal effect on *S. aureus* mediated by NET is dependent on the activity of MPO. Similarly, antifungal activity of NETs has been assigned to zinc chelating cation calgranulin, which is required for fungal growth (Pilsczek et al., 2010). Histones can restrict microbial growth very proficiently, and antibodies against histones prevent NET-mediated microbicidal activity (Brinkmann et al., 2004). The entrapment of microbes takes place due to the electrostatic interactions between the positively charged bacterial surface and the negatively charged chromatin fibers (Brinkmann & Zychlinsky, 2007). This entrapment can be evaded by encapsulated pathogens or those that can change their surface charge (Wartha et al., 2007). Importantly, by the help of nucleases, several bacteria are able to degrade NETs and thus escape NET-mediated entrapment, which include the Gram-negative pathogen *Vibrium cholera* and the Gram-positive bacteria *Streptococcus pneumoniae*, *S. pyogenes*, *Yersinia* sp., *Streptococcus agalactiae*, *Streptococcus suis*, *S. aureus*, and *Aeromonas hydrophila* (Yang & Biermann, 2016). This underlines the significance of nucleases as pathogenic factors.

Different species of bacteria, viruses, fungi, and parasites, associate with a variety of NET-mediated inflammatory processes. A brief description of species-wise antimicrobial NET activity has been provided further.

Bacteria

Staphylococcus aureus

Chiefly residing in wet squamous epithelium of the anterior nasal cavity in the human body, *S. aureus* is a Gram-positive bacterium often known as a "super bacterium" due to its ability to evade immune responses and resist antibiotic treatment. It causes pathologies such as, bacteraemia, endocarditis, osteomyelitis, and gastroenteritis, which are associated with severe inflammatory response (Liu, 2009). *S. aureus* was initially used as an inducer of NETosis in classic assays performed by Brinkmann et al. (2004). Pilsczek et al. (2010) discovered that *S. aureus* led to a notably faster NETosis that was independent of ROS, which they named "vital NETosis," when inducing NET formation and studying its molecular mechanisms (Pilsczek et al., 2015). *S. aureus* evades host immune system by secretion of numerous virulence factors, such as Panton—Valentine leucocidin (PVL), leukotoxin DE, leukotoxin GH (LukGH), N-terminal ArgD peptides, and gamma-hemolysin, of which LukGH and PVL stimulate NETs through an oxidative pathway-independent mechanism (Gonzalez et al., 2014; Malachowa, Kobayashi, Freedman, Dorward, & DeLeo, 2013; Pilsczek et al., 2015). NET formation is promoted by bacterial invasion which traps pathogens and obstructs their spread. Macrophages through phagocytosis and cytokine production support this innate immune response. According to reports, *S. aureus* may have a cytotoxic effect on macrophages through these NETs, since NET incubation with nucleases and adenosine synthases derived from this bacterium promotes the formation of deoxy-adenosine, which is capable of inducing cell death (Tammavongsa, Missiakas, & Schneewind, 2014).

Streptococcus pneumoniae

It can be typically found in the human respiratory tract, *S. pneumoniae* is a Gram-positive bacterium whose role in NET induction has been well instituted (Brinkmann et al., 2004). Comparable to *S. aureus*, *S. pneumoniae* can produce virulence factors such as endA which digests DNA, allowing it to escape from NETs even after bacteria have been trapped in it. This promotes bacteria dissemination from upper respiratory tract to the lungs and then to the bloodstream (Beiter et al., 2006; Moorthy et al., 2016; Zhu, Kuang, Wilson, & Lau, 2013). NETosis has also been associated in the progression and complications of respiratory diseases due to secondary infections such as chronic obstructive pulmonary disease, pneumonia, and emphysema (Bass et al., 2010; Moorthy et al., 2013; Young et al., 2011). Neutrophils disrupt microcirculation and induce more NETosis in pulmonary alveoli when excessively recruited to lung tissue in response to infection. Additionally, patients with pulmonary dysfunction show elevated levels of extracellular DNA than patients with mild lung disease, showing that NETs participate in airflow obstruction and extend chronic inflammatory responses (Dworski, Simon, Hoskins, & Yousef, 2011; Pedersen et al., 2015).

Escherichia coli

Escherichia coli is the most abundant facultative anaerobe among the host microbiota, a Gram-negative bacterium that inhabits in the human gastrointestinal tract at birth (Kaper, Nataro, & Mobley, 2004). It has been involved in pathologies such as enteritis, urinary infections, meningitis, and sepsis (Croxen & Finlay, 2010). Finally, Kambas et al. (2012) found that in *E. coli* infected serum of patients with septic shock, when neutrophils are stimulated NETs are significantly induced. This might be probably through the stimulation of TLRs or complement receptors for C3 or C5a (Kambas et al., 2012). Several studies report that NETs and their components aggravate septicemia (Daigo et al., 2012; Seeley, Matthay, & Wolters, 2012; Tanaka et al.,2014), since their degradation with DNases alongside antibiotic treatment diminishes tissue damage (Czaikoski et al., 2016). Neutrophils are adept in distinguishing between LPS from diverse pathogens and strains in order to induce NET formation and release tissue factor, thrombogen that has been involved in systemic inflammatory responses facilitated by initiation of the coagulation system that typifies septic processes (Fuchs et al., 2010; Pieterse, Rother, Yanginlar, Hilbrands, & van der Vlag, 2016). Cells of the urinary tract are not able to eliminate infections caused by *E. coli* as concentrations of the AMP, LL37, is high. Nevertheless, LL37 considerably decreases bacterial colonization (Chromek et al., 2006) as it is associated with NETs (Brinkmann et al., 2004) and supports their formation and stability (Neumann et al., 2014).

Clostridium difficile

Clostridium difficile is the strain of bacteria that causes diarrhea and pseudomembranous colitis in humans, mostly due to the abuse of antibiotics (Garey, Sethi, Yadav, & DuPont, 2008) that strictly harms the host resident microbiota, leading to dysbiosis (Lange, Buerger, Stallmach, & Bruns, 2016). *C. difficile* is the normal component of the human microbiota which cannot reproduce excessively as compared to other resident species because of its competition with those species (Kopke, Straub, & Durre, 2013). Conversely, alteration of the microbiota increases nutrient availability along with the moderated production of secondary biliary acids, which allows for *C. difficile* colonization of the gut (Sorg & Sonenshein, 2010). *C. difficile* causes the loss of tight junctions and is able to translocate through the ability of its enterotoxins. Upon contact with cells of the gut-associated lymphoid tissue, proinflammatory cytokines production is promoted and chemokines such as interleukin 1 beta (IL-1β), IL-8, and CXCL5 are promoted for the recruitment of neutrophils (Nusrat et al., 2001). Neutrophils do not merely reduce the function of microbial toxins by exuding AMPs and elastase, but also ejects NETs, which cover the injured areas of the intestinal epithelium to effectually thwart *C. difficile* dissemination.

Shigella flexneri

Shigella flexneri is an enteropathogenic bacterium whose infection may cause dysentery in the host. This is a Gram-negative bacterium usually acquired by the ingestion of contaminated food and beverages. *Shigella* can navigate the intestinal lumen across M cells; once there, it infects epithelial cells and may spread in parallel. As a result of which, nuclear factor kappa B (NF-κB) is activated in infected cells, which produce IL-8 to draw neutrophils to infected tissues, where neutrophil-derived elastase degrades microbial virulence factors (Eilers et al., 2010; Phalipon & Sansonetti, 2007). As reported by Brinkmann et al. (2004), *S. flexneri* is trapped within NETs in vitro and has the ability of DNA-associated elastase to degrade the virulence factors IcsA and IpaB. It was also showed that in zones with severe neutrophil infiltration, in vitro neutrophil transmigration is required for *Shigella* invasion and pathogenesis (Perdomo, Gounon, & Sansonetti, 1994).

Salmonella typhimurium

Salmonella, a genus of facultative anaerobic intracellular bacteria and many species of this genus can be found in the gut microbiota. *S. typhimurium* is a leading cause of infectious gastroenteritis. After taking possession in the gut, it can enter into enterocytes, M cells, dendritic cells (DCs), and, finally, into macrophages upon reaching the submucosa. It typically replicates inside phagosomes where it may express several virulence factors such as adhesins, flagella, fimbriae, and T3SS (Griffin & McSorley, 2011). Using a SOD known as SodCl, it is also capable of counteracting the activity of ROS in the phagosome of leukocytes (Ibarra & Steele-Mortimer, 2009; Pacello et al., 2008).

Brinkmann et al. (2004) have showed that *S. typhimurium* also stimulates NETs. They have also shown that it is effectively trapped and eliminated by components of NETs, including granular proteins and H2A histone (Brinkmann et al., 2004).

Yersinia enterocolitica

Y. enterocolitica is the underlying agent of yersiniosis, acute enteritis, and enterocolitis. It annexes the epithelium and translocates to Peyer's patches and affects tight junctions by diminishing occludin and claudins 5 and 8 (Hering et al., 2016). All three pathogenic species of *Yersinia*, namely, *Y. pseudotuberculosis*, *Y. enterocolitica*, and *Y. pestis*, mainly aim to translocate their effector proteins (known as Yops) into neutrophils, macrophages, and DCs. Furthermore *Y. pestis* hinders the oxidative burst of neutrophils in order to support its own intracellular survival using Yops proteins (Spinner et al., 2010).

Mollerherm et al. (2015) proved that serotypes 0:3, 0:8, and 0:8 of *Y. entero-colitica* induce NETs in vitro within 1 hour of incubation. However, with increasing time, NET induction was diminished suggesting that Ca^{++}- and Mg^{++}-dependent nucleases may hinder NETosis (Mollerherm et al., 2015). By employing a special protein called invasin, *Y. pseudotuberculosis* can breach the intestinal epithelium. Invasin is a highly adhesive protein that mediates binding of M cells to the $\beta1$ integrins in *Y. pseudotuberculosis*, though this binding induces ROS production and NET formation.

Mycobacterium tuberculosis

M. tuberculosis is an obligate aerobic bacterium that causes tuberculosis. It stands out amongst the best intracellular pathogens in regard to its techniques for avoidance of the immune system. Principally, it infects the respiratory system, but may also affect other organs. Its cell envelope comprises of adhesins and, in comparison to other pathogenic bacteria, it does not produce toxins. For replication and dissemination throughout the host organism, it uses phagocytes. On coculturing with neutrophils of different genotypes, it has been shown that it induces NETs. Although NETs effectively trap and obstruct the dissemination of mycobacteria, they are not killed by NET-derived components (Ramos-Kichik et al., 2009). *M. tuberculosis* augments the apoptosis of neutrophils to stop them from creating granulomas as a mechanism of immune evasion, which are structures comprising of immune cells in response to primary infection, to restrain this bacillus. Macrophage efferocytosis of apoptotic neutrophils has a proinflammatory effect in immune response. In apoptotic and necrotic cells (Persson, Blomgran-Julinder, Rahman, Zheng, & Stendahl, 2008) and in DNA within NETs, heat shock protein 72 has been found which also plays necessary role in the elimination of *M. tuberculosis* (Braian, Hogea, & Stendahl, 2013).

Vibrio cholerae

This species is widely renowned because of cholera pandemics provoked by the O1 and O139 serogroups. *Vibrio cholerae* is a Gram-negative bacterium and is generally found in the human gastrointestinal tract and in aquatic environments; seemingly, infections usually ensue due to the ingestion of contaminated seafood and water. On reaching the gut, *V. cholerae* secretes cholera toxin as well as adhesins, hemagglutinin, proteases, and hemolysins. Lastly, *V. cholerae* stimulates neutrophil recruitment to the gut and the production of cytokines (Reidl & Klose, 2002). There are reports that upon contact with neutrophils in vitro, *V. cholerae* induced NETs. However, nucleases Dns and Xds are secreted by *V. cholera* as an evasion mechanism that allows it to escape from NETs, thus letting it continue the infectious process. Therefore *V. cholerae* infection does not have a protection mechanism in NETs (Seper et al., 2013).

Lactobacillus rhamnosus

Lactobacillus rhamnosus is a Gram-positive bacterium that has been primarily studied for its capacities to restore the intestinal barrier, hence deemed as an essential probiotic for the microbiota. It is able to cling to the intestinal epithelium and to endure gastric acid and bile (Doron, Snydman, & Gorbach, 2005). It reduces the epithelial injury caused by ulcerative colitis and Crohn's disease (CD) (Zigra, Maipa, & Alamanos, 2007). *L. rhamnosus* stimulates TLRs on immune cells to modulate the immune response and intestinal microbiota (Ginsburg, 2002). It has been shown that upon induction by other microbes (*S. aureus* and *E. coli*) or chemicals (phorbol-12-myristate-13-acetate, better known as PMA), *L. rhamnosus* inhibits NET formation, possibly due to its antioxidant activity and yet unknown secreted proteins.

Viruses

Influenza

Influenza A virus is a deadly virus known for killing over 50 million people in 1918 and, lately for the 2009 pandemics accountable for 18,000 deaths around the world. Influenza pathology is described by excessive recruitment of neutrophils to the lungs, which is aided by chemokine receptor 2 (CXCR2). Influenza A-stimulated NETs are dependent on PAD4 (Hemmers, Teijaro, Arandjelovic, & Mowen, 2011). Through the blockage of the PKC pathway α-Defensin-1 associated with NETs inhibits virus replication. Another component which stimulates influenza A virus for bactericidal NETs is, LL37 which has been shown to increase NET production in response to this pathogen in vitro (Tripathi, Verma, Kim, White, & Hartshorn, 2014). Moreover viral aggregation and neutralization requires arginine-rich H3 and H4 histones. Incubation of influenza A virus with H4 has revealed a major decrease in viral replication in epithelial cells; by contrast, H4 was put out of action when incubated with the pandemic strain H1N1, which may emphasize its importance in response to this pathogen (Hoeksema et al., 2015). The disadvantage of disproportionate neutrophil infiltration includes injury to tissues facilitated by AMPs and extensive NETs in the alveolar capillaries (Dworski et al., 2011; Pedersen et al., 2015).

Dengue virus (DENV)

It is a single-stranded RNA virus that has several dengue serotypes with outcomes that span from mild fever to severe dengue, formerly known as dengue hemorrhagic fever (Moreno-Altamirano, Rodriguez-Espinosa, Rojas-Espinosa, PliegoRivero, & Sanchez-Garcia, 2015). It belongs to the Flaviviridae family. In recent years the incidence of dengue infections has increased; therefore, understanding the mechanisms of host defense used to fight this pathogen is necessary. By trapping viruses within their structures,

NETs can restrain infections. However, it has been reported that rather than inducing NETs, DENV-2 inhibits them in vitro. As observed by Moreno-Altamirano et al. (2015), there is an 80% decrease in PMA-stimulated NET formation by neutrophils following previous incubation with DENV-1. This inhibition was caused by the disruption of a chief metabolic requirement for NET release (Rodriguez-Espinosa, Rojas-Espinosa, Moreno-Altamirano, LopezVillegas, & Sanchez-Garcia, 2015) that is glut-1-mediated glucose uptake (Moreno-Altamirano et al., 2015).

Human immunodeficiency virus 1

Human immunodeficiency virus 1 (HIV-1) is an immune system affecting virus. Currently over 35 million people are infected, with about 2 million being infected every year (Kaminski et al., 2016). It has been reported that the receptor for virus entry is CD4, along with CCR5 and CXCR4, which permits not only the infection of CD4 T cells but also antigen-presenting cells such as macrophages and DCs. However, activated T cells wherein viral replication takes place quickly and efficiently, produce most of the serum. TLR7 and TLR8 pathways help in the recognition of HIV-1-derived nucleic acids in neutrophils. Subsequently they liberate ROS in order to stimulate NET formation. Through the action of MPO and α-defensins, to both of which antiviral activity has been attributed to, NET structures may trap, contain, and eliminate HIV. HIV, as an immune evasion mechanism, elevates IL-10 production by DCs, thus preventing ROS and NET release (Saitoh et al., 2012).

Respiratory syncytial virus

Respiratory syncytial virus (RSV) is one of the most important pediatric infections and leading cause of hospitalization in 1-year-old infants. RSV triggers acute bronchitis, mucosal and submucosal edema, and luminal occlusion by cellular debris formed from epithelial cells, macrophages, fibrin strands, and mucin. By infecting DCs, RSV diminishes their antigen-presenting capacity to activate T cells (Borchers, Chang, Gershwin, & Gershwin, 2013). RSVs may release NETs in vitro by stimulating neutrophils, as shown in samples of bronchoalveolar lavage fluid from patients with severe disease of the lower respiratory tract caused by RSV. RSV dissemination is prevented due to NET formation, but these NETs are unable to kill the virus (Cortjens et al.,2016). Moreover by TLR4 pathway RSV F-protein is also able to induce NETs. The presence of NETs may aggravate inflammatory symptoms and promote luminal occlusion with structures composed of mucus and DNA despite acting as viral reservoirs (Funchal et al., 2015).

Fungi

Candida albicans

C. albicans typically causes disease only in immunocompromised subjects, such as patients on antibiotic treatment or with a central venous catheter, patients with pancreatitis or renal insufficiency, and in patients following gastrointestinal surgery. But is usually found colonizing the mucosa, skin, and oral cavity in healthy individuals, Morphological transformation of yeast to hyphae as exemplified by *C. albicans* produces several virulence factors such as Als (Brinkmann et al., 2004) and Ssa invasins (Mulcahy, Charron-Mazenod, & Lewenza, 2008), which act as invasive pathogens. Recognition of *C. albicans* by epithelial cells and macrophages releases chemokines that attract neutrophils (Mayer, Wilson, & Hube, 2013; Netea, Joosten, van der Meer, Kullberg, & van de Veerdonk, 2015). By releasing NETs in either its yeast or hyphal form, neutrophils are able to trap and eliminate *C. albicans* (Urban et al., 2006). To succeed a fast NETosis response, the β-glucan on hyphae must be recognized by CR3, and fibronectin, a component of the extracellular matrix, must be present. These elements are required for homotypic cellular aggregation supported by NETs, but are independent of ROS production (Byrd, Obrien, Johnson, Lavigne, & Reichner, 2013).

Aspergillus fumigatus

In healthy humans *A. fumigatus* is a part of the human microbiota. It causes invasive aspergillosis in immunosuppressed individuals, and is accountable for a leading mycotic infection in patients with CGD by both prevalence and mortality rate (Segal & Romani, 2009). Inhalation of spores infects the immune system cells, which instead of being eliminated, ends by residing in the respiratory tract with an altered morphology from yeast to hyphae, infecting the lungs causing pneumonia and infection of other organs. It produces invasins similar to *C. albicans* that allow it to cling to the host cells (Askew, 2009; Lee et al., 2015). NETs release upon induction by *A. fumigatus* in vitro entails activation of NOX (Bianchi et al., 2009). Additionally, deletion of p46(−/−) in mice deters NET formation (Rohm et al., 2014). Even though NETs are essential for the arrest and abolition of *A. fumigatus* hyphae, these are not caused by spores as Rod A present in the spore cell wall (Bruns et al., 2010).

Cryptococcus spp.

Cryptococcus neoformans is a pathogenic yeast which causes diseases like cryptococcosis and meningoencephalitis. Infection results after spores are breathe in which enters the alveolar space, whereby they stay dormant until immunological instability occurs (Bose, Reese, Ory, Janbon, & Doering, 2003). A capsular polysaccharide present in *C. neoformans* bestows its host immune system regulating ability. Specifically, it is able to restrain production of NETs. Capsules in strains enclosing glucuronoxylomannan (GXM) and galactoxylomannan in neutrophils were not effective producers of either ROS or NETs, even after stimulation with PMA. Upon incubation of neutrophils with strains without capsular GXM, NETs were effectually produced; however, ROS production was not noted. Thus capsular GXM mediates resistance to NETs by improving virulence. Lastly NET-associated AMPs, such as elastase, MPO, collagenase, and histones, have microbial activity required to kill this pathogen (Rocha et al., 2015).

Parasites

Plasmodium falciparum

Plasmodium falciparum is the underlying means of malaria, renowned as paludism. It strictly affects children below 5 years old, who denote 90% of deaths associated with this disease (Chan, Fowkes, & Beeson, 2014). Malaria is a blood vector-borne disease transmitted by mosquitoes. *Plasmodium* sp. induces the production of inflammatory cytokines by infecting erythrocytes, suppressing erythropoiesis and leading to anemia. Invasion is facilitated by proteins on affected erythrocytes that stimulate their adhesion to the vascular endothelium present in tissue and organs and invoke an inflammatory response and coagulation. This process of infection triggers vascular damage, abrasions on endothelial cells, and activation of platelets, monocytes, and neutrophils. NETs can be found in the circulation of *P. falciparum* infected children with *P. falciparum* adhering to erythrocytes and parasites. Moreover α-dsDNA antibodies discovered in these patients may participate in the progression of this pathology, exacerbating the immune response and autoimmune processes (Baker et al., 2008). Conversely antihemostatic agaphelin produced by the glands of infected mosquitoes impede neutrophil chemotaxis, obstruct aggregation of platelets facilitated by cathepsin/elastase, and diminish neutrophil-induced coagulation (Waisberg et al., 2014).

Toxoplasma gondii

Toxoplasma gondii, infecting over a third of the population worldwide, is the causal agent of toxoplasmosis, which occurs as a result of the ingestion of contaminated food. *T. gondii* infection stimulates recruitment of neutrophils to the infected site (Nathan, 2006). Fittingly, in a murine model of intranasal infection, dissemination of this pathogen is limited by neutrophils, trapping it and killing it in NETs, thus indicating that active incursion is not obligatory for NET formation. This observation was later revealed in humans, further disclosing that NET formation is dependent on MEK−ERK (Abdallah, Lin, Ball, King, Duhamel, & Denkers, 2012).

NETosis and cytokines

Cytokines are small proteins ($\sim 5-20$ kDa) secreted by cells of the immune system that mediates various effects on other cells. These are categorized into three broad categories—interferon, interleukin, and growth factors. These signaling proteins regulate a spectrum of biological operations including innate and acquired immunity, hematopoiesis, inflammation and repair, and proliferation through mostly extracellular signaling. Secreted by several cell types at local high concentration, cytokines mediate cell-to-cell interaction, have regulating effects on nearby cells and henceforth, function mostly in paracrine fashion. These polypeptides also act as cell distress signals that recruit immune cells like neutrophils to the site of immune injury. Through their release into the circulation (endocrine or systemic effect) cytokines may exert their effects on distant cells or may do so in the secreting cell itself (autocrine effect). Cytokines also lead to postponement of apoptosis of neutrophil, a process important for regulation of host resistance and inflammation (Colotta, Re, Polentarutti, Sozzani, & Mantovani, 1992).

In NETosis various cytokines function as mediators of inflammatory processes and the mechanisms by which they act are mostly unknown. IL-6 and TNF-α act as circulating biomarkers of NETosis. Together with TNF-α and macrophage migration-inhibitory factor, they act as inflammatory mediators to alter microvascular homeostasis (Dinarello, 1997; Feghali & Wright, 1997; Fortin, McDonald, Fulop, & Lesur, 2010; Wu, Tyml, & Wilson, 2008) in blood flow and have been associated with multiple organ dysfunction syndrome. Induction of NETs in macrophages leads to the activation of inflammasome and subsequent secretion of proinflammatory cytokines IL-1β and IL-18 (Kahlenberg Carmona-Rivera, Smith, & Kaplan, 2013). Secreted IL-1β and IL-18 induce NET formation, forming a feedback loop as reported in the pathogenesis of SLE (Kahlenberg et al., 2013; Mitroulis et al., 2011). MSU crystals trigger release of IL-1β derived from macrophages which enhances NET release. Recombinant IL-1β amplifies superoxide production and spreading of PMNs by priming human PMNs for MPO release (Dularay, Elson, Clements-Jewery, Damais, & Lando, 1990).

Similar to PMA and LPS, IL-8 also induces NET formation. IL-8 induces elastase release in a concentration-dependent manner in cytochalasin B−treated PMNs and IL-1β was found to prime this release (Brandolini, Bertini, Bizzarri, Sergi, & Caselli, 1996). By targeting PMNs and stimulating PMN adhesion, degranulation, respiratory burst, and lipid mediator synthesis, IL-8 contributes to NETosis (Baggiolini, Dewald, & Moser, 1994). Neutralization of IL-8 using antibody has been found to prevent tissue damage in NET-induced diseases such as glomerulonephritis (Harada, Sekido, Akahoshi, Wada, & Mukaida, 1994).

Recombinant forms of human TNF-α considerably raised neutrophil respiratory response to N-formylmethionine-leucyl-phenylalanine (fMLP) while stimulating neutrophil respiratory and lysozyme release (Ferrante, Nandoskar, Walz, Goh, & Kowanko, 1988). By increasing phagocytosis, degranulation and oxidative burst is seen in bovine PMNs, TNF-α enhanced migration within endothelium conferred due to elevation of endothelial adhesion molecules (Paape, Bannerman, Zhao, & Lee, 2003). These mediators regulate generation of cytokines in PMNs, such as addition of nitric oxide augments TNF-α secretion from human neutrophils (Van Dervort, Yan, Madara, Cobb, & Wesley, 1994).

Type I interferons which play a major role in SLE pathogenesis elicit differentiation of plasmacytoid DCs from monocytes upon interacting with NET autoantigens. In addition to nuclear DNA, mitochondrial DNA (mtDNA) deposition has been found in NETs in renal biopsy specimen of lupus nephritis. These mtDNA have greater propensity of triggering IFN α production from peripheral DCs via TLRs than that of dsDNA/antidsDNA.

In addition to these cytokines, interlukin-17A (IL-17A), a proinflammatory cytokine secreted by Th-17 help T cell, activates the recruitment of innate immune cells. In psoriasis a chronic skin condition caused by an overactive immune system, mast cells and neutrophils predominantly secrete IL-17 at greater densities and form specialized structures called extracellular traps. Thus cytokines play key roles in both induction and continuation of NETosis by regulating various cellular processes.

References

Abdallah, D. S. A., Lin, C., Ball, C. J., King, M. R., Duhamel, G. E., & Denkers, E. Y. (2012). Toxoplasma gondii triggers release of human and mouse neutrophil extracellular traps. *Infection and Immunity, 80*, 768−777.

Allam, R., Kumar, S. V., Darisipudi, M. N., & Anders, H. J. (2014). Extracellular histones in tissue injury and inflammation. *Journal of Molecular Medicine, 92*, 465−467.

Amini, P., Stojkov, D., Wang, X., Wicki, S., Kaufmann, T., Wong, W. W., & Yousefi, S. (2016). NET formation can occur independently of RIPK3 and MLKL signaling. *European journal of immunology, 46*, 178−184.

Amulic, B., Knackstedt, S. L., Abu Abed, U., Deigendesch, N., Harbort, C. J., Caffrey, B. E., ... Zychlinsky, A. (2017). Cell-cycle proteins control production of neutrophil extracellular traps. *Developmental Cell, 43*, 449−462.

Askew, D. S. (2009). Aspergillus fumigatus: Virulence genes in a street-smart mold. *Current Opinion in Microbiology, 11*, 331−337. Available from https://doi.org/10.1016/j.mib.2008.05.009.

Aulik, N. A., Hellenbrand, K. M., Klos, H., & Czuprynski, C. J. (2010). Mannheimia haemolytica and its leukotoxin cause neutrophil extracellular trap formation by bovine neutrophils. *Infection and Immunity, 78*, 4454−4466.

Averhoff, P., Kolbe, M., Zychlinsky, A., & Weinrauch, Y. (2008). Single residue determines the specificity of neutrophil elastase for Shigella virulence factors. *Journal of Molecular Biology, 377*, 1053−1066.

Babior, B. M. (1999). NADPH oxidase: An update. *Blood, 93*, 1464−1476.

Baggiolini, M., Dewald, B., & Moser, B. (1994). Interleukin-8 and related chemotactic cytokines−CXC and CC chemokines. *Advances in Immunology, 55*, 97−179.

Baker, V. S., Imade, G. E., Molta, N. B., Tawde, P., Pam, S. D., & Obadofn, M. O. (2008). Cytokine-associated neutrophil extracellular traps and antinuclear antibodies in *Plasmodium falciparum* infected children under six years of age. *Malaria Journal*, *7*, 41. Available from https://doi.org/10.1186/1475-2875-7-41.

Bannister, A. J., & Kouzarides, T. (2011). Regulation of chromatin by histone modifications. *Cell Research*, *21*, 381–395.

Bass, J. I. F., Russo, D. M., Gabelloni, M. L., Geffner, J. R., Giordano, M., & Catalano, M. (2010). Extracellular DNA: A major proinflammatory component of *Pseudomonas aeruginosa* bioflms. *Journal of Immunology*, *184*, 6386–6395. Available from https://doi.org/10.4049/jimmunol.0901640.

Beaudouin, J., Gerlich, D., Daigle, N., Eils, R., & Ellenberg, J. (2002). Nuclear envelope breakdown proceeds by microtubule-induced tearing of the lamina. *Cell.*, *108*, 83–96.

Beiter, K., Wartha, F., Albiger, B., Normark, S., Zychlinsky, A., & Henriques-Normark, B. (2006). An endonuclease allows *Streptococcus pneumoniae* to escape from neutrophil extracellular traps. *Current Biology*, *16*, 401–407. Available from https://doi.org/10.1016/j.cub.2006.01.056.

Bhattacharya, A., Wei, Q., Shin, J. N., Abdel, F. E., Bonilla, D. L., Xiang, Q., & Eissa, N. T. (2015). Autophagy Is Required for Neutrophil-Mediated Inflammation. *Cell Reports*, *12*, 1731–1739.

Bianchi, M., Hakkim, A., Brinkmann, V., Siler, U., Seger, R. A., Zychlinsky, A., & Reichenbach, J. (2009). Restoration of NET formation by gene therapy in CGD controls aspergillosis. *Blood*, *114*, 2619–2622.

Borchers, A. T., Chang, C., Gershwin, M. E., & Gershwin, L. J. (2013). Respiratory syncytial virus − A comprehensive review. *Clinical Reviews in Allergy Immunology*, *45*, 331–379. Available from https://doi.org/10.1007/s12016-013-8368-9.

Bose, I., Reese, A. J., Ory, J. J., Janbon, G., & Doering, T. L. (2003). A yeast under cover: The capsule of *Cryptococcus neoformans*. *Eukaryotic Cell*, *2*, 655–663. Available from https://doi.org/10.1128/EC.2.4.655-663.2003.

Braian, C., Hogea, V., & Stendahl, O. (2013). Mycobacterium tuberculosis-induced neutrophil extracellular traps activate human macrophages. *Journal of Innate Immunology*, *5*, 591–602. Available from https://doi.org/10.1159/000348676.

Brandolini, L., Bertini, R., Bizzarri, C., Sergi, R., & Caselli, G. (1996). IL-1 beta primes IL-8-activated human neutrophils for elastase release, phospholipase D activity, and calcium flux. *Journal of Leukocyte Biology*, *59*, 427–434.

Branzk, N., et al. (2014). Neutrophils sense microbe size and selectively release neutrophil extracellular traps in response to large pathogens. *Nature Immunology*, *15*, 1017–1025.

Brinkmann, V., Reichard, U., Goosmann, C., Fauler, B., Uhlemann, Y., Weiss, D. S., ... Zychlinsky, A. (2004). Neutrophil extracellular traps kill bacteria. *Science*, *303*, 1532–1535.

Brinkmann, V., & Zychlinsky, A. (2007). Beneficial suicide: Why neutrophils die to make NETs. *Nature Reviews Microbiology*, *5*, 577–582.

Bruns, S., Kniemeyer, O., Hasenberg, M., Aimanianda, V., Nietzsche, S., & Tywissen, A. (2010). Production of extracellular traps against *Aspergillus fumigatus* in vitro and in infected lung tissue is dependent on invading neutrophils and influenced by hydrophobin RodA. *PLoS Pathogens*, *6*, e1000873. Available from https://doi.org/10.1371/journal.ppat.1000873.

Byrd, A. S., Obrien, X. M., Johnson, C. M., Lavigne, L. M., & Reichner, J. S. (2013). An extracellular matrix-based mechanism of rapid neutrophil extracellular trap formation in response to *Candida albicans*. *Journal of Immunology*, *190*, 4136–4148. Available from https://doi.org/10.4049/jimmunol.1202671.

Chan, J. A., Fowkes, F. J., & Beeson, J. G. (2014). Surface antigens of *Plasmodium falciparum*-infected erythrocytes as immune targets and malaria vaccine candidates. *Cellular and Molecular Life Science*, *71*, 3633−3657. Available from https://doi.org/10.1007/s00018-014-1614-3.

Chen, K. W., Monteleone1, M., Boucher, D., Sollberger, G., Ramnath, D., Condon, N. D., . . . Schroder, K. (2018). Noncanonical inflammasome signaling elicits gasdermin D−dependent neutrophil extracellular traps*Science Immunology*, pii: eaar6676. Available from https://doi.org/10.1126/sciimmunol.aar6676.

Chromek, M., Slamova, Z., Bergman, P., Kovacs, L., Podracka, L., & Ehren, I. (2006). The antimicrobial peptide cathelicidin protects the urinary tract against invasive bacterial infection. *Nature Medicine*, *12*, 636−641. Available from https://doi.org/10.1038/nm1407.

Clark, S. R., Ma, A. C., Tavener, S. A., McDonald, B., Goodarzi, Z., Kelly, M. M., . . . Kubes, P. (2007). Platelet TLR4 activates neutrophil extracellular traps to ensnare bacteria in septic blood. *Nature Medicine*, *13*, 463469.

Colotta, F., Re, F., Polentarutti, N., Sozzani, S., & Mantovani, A. (1992). Modulation of granulocyte survival and programmed cell death by cytokines and bacterial products. *Blood*, *80*, 2012−2020.

Cools-Lartigue, J., Spicer, J., & McDonald, B. (2013). Neutrophil extracellular traps sequester circulating tumor cells and promote metastasis. *Journal of Clinical Investigation*. Available from https://doi.org/10.1172/JCI67484.

Cortjens, B., de Boer, O. J., de Jong, R., Antonis, A. F., Sabogal, P. Y. S., & Lutter, R. (2016). Neutrophil extracellular traps cause airway obstruction during respiratory syncytial virus disease. *Journal of Pathology*, *238*, 401−411. Available from https://doi.org/10.1002/path.4660.

Croxen, M. A., & Finlay, B. B. (2010). Molecular mechanisms of *Escherichia coli* pathogenicity. *Nature Reviews Microbiology*, *8*, 26−38. Available from https://doi.org/10.1038/nrmicro2265.

Czaikoski, P. G., Mota, J. M., Nascimento, D. C., Sonego, F., Castanheira, F. V., & Melo, P. H. (2016). Neutrophil extracellular traps induce organ damage during experimental and clinical sepsis. *PLoS One*, *11*, e0148142. Available from https://doi.org/10.1371/journal.pone.0148142.

Daigo, K., Yamaguchi, N., Kawamura, T., Matsubara, K., Jiang, S., & Ohashi, R. (2012). The proteomic profile of circulating pentraxin 3 (PTX3) complex in sepsis demonstrates the interaction with azurocidin 1 and other components of neutrophil extracellular traps. *Molecular and Cell Proteomics*, *11*. Available from https://doi.org/10.1074/mcp.M111.015073, M111.015073.

Delbosc, S., Alsac, J. M., Journe, C., Louedec, L., Castier, Y., & Bonnaure-Mallet, M. (2011). *Porphyromonas gingivalis* participates in pathogenesis of human abdominal aortic aneurysm by neutrophil activation: Proof of concept in rats. *PLoS One*, *6*(4), e18679. Available from https://doi.org/10.1371/journal.pone.0018679.

Desai, J., Kumar, S. V., Mulay, S. R., Konrad, L., Romoli, S., Schauer, C., . . . Anders, H. J. (2016). PMA and crystal-induced neutrophil extracellular trap formation involves RIPK1-RIPK3-MLKL signaling. *European Journal of Immunology*, *49*, 223−229.

Dinarello, C. A. (1997). Proinflammatory and anti-inflammatory cytokines as mediators in the pathogenesis of septic shock. *Chest*, *112*, 321S−329S.

Dinauer, M. C. (2003). Regulation of neutrophil function by Rac GTPases. *Current Opinion in Hematology*, *10*, 8−15.

Doron, S., Snydman, D. R., & Gorbach, S. L. (2005). Lactobacillus GG: Bacteriology and clinical applications. *Gastroenterology Clinics North America*, *34*, 483−498. Available from https://doi.org/10.1016/j.gtc.2005.05.011.

Dularay, B., Elson, C. J., Clements-Jewery, S., Damais, C., & Lando, D. (1990). Recombinant human interleukin-1 beta primes human polymorphonuclear leukocytes for stimulus-induced myeloperoxidase release. *Journal of Leukocyte Biology*, *47*, 158−163.

Dwivedi, N., Neeli, I., Schall, N., Wan, H., Desiderio, D. M., Csernok, E., . . . Muller, S. (2014). Deimination of linker histones links neutrophil extracellular trap release with autoantibodies in systemic autoimmunity. *Federation of American Societies for Experimental Biology Journal*, *28*, 2840−2851.

Dworski, R., Simon, H. U., Hoskins, A., & Yousef, S. (2011). Eosinophil and neutrophil extracellular DNA traps in human allergic asthmatic airways. *Journal of Allergy and Clinical Immunology*, *127*, 1260−1266. Available from https://doi.org/10.1016/j.jaci.2010.12.1103.

Eilers, B., Mayer-Scholl, A., Walker, T., Tang, C., Weinrauch, Y., & Zychlinsky, A. (2010). Neutrophil antimicrobial proteins enhance *Shigella flexneri* adhesion and invasion. *Cell Microbiology*, *12*, 1134−1143. Available from https://doi.org/10.1111/j.1462-5822.2010.01459.

Farquharson, D., Butcher, J. P., & Culshaw, S. (2012). Periodontitis, porphyromonas, and the pathogenesis of rheumatoid arthritis. *Mucosal Immunology*, *5*, 112120.

Feghali, C. A., & Wright, T. M. (1997). Cytokines in acute and chronic inflammation. *Frontiers in Bioscience*, *2*, d12−d26.

Ferrante, A., Nandoskar, M., Walz, A., Goh, D. H., & Kowanko, I. C. (1988). Effects of tumour necrosis factor alpha and interleukin-1 alpha and beta on human neutrophil migration, respiratory burst and degranulation. *International Archives of Allergy and Immunology*, *86*, 82−91.

Filomeni, G., De Zio, D., & Cecconi, F. (2015). Oxidative stress and autophagy: the clash between damage and metabolic needs. *Cell Death and Differentiation*, *22*, 377−388.

Fortin, C. F., McDonald, P. P., Fulop, T., & Lesur, O. (2010). Sepsis, leukocytes, and nitric oxide (NO): An intricate affair. *Shock*, *33*, 344−352.

Fuchs, T. A., Abed, U., Goosmann, C., Hurwitz, R., Schulze, I., & Wahn, V. (2007). Novel cell death program leads to neutrophil extracellular traps. *Journal of Cell Biology*, *176*, 231−241.

Fuchs, T. A., Brill, A., & Duerschmied, D. (2010). Extracellular DNA traps promote thrombosis. *Proceedings of the National Academy of Sciences of the United States of America*, *107*, 15880−15885.

Funchal, G. A., Jaeger, N., Czepielewski, R. S., Machado, M. S., Muraro, S. P., & Stein, R. T. (2015). Respiratory syncytial virus fusion protein promotes TLR-4-dependent neutrophil extracellular trap formation by human neutrophils. *PLoS One*, *10*, e0124082. Available from https://doi.org/10.1371/journal.pone.0124082.

Garcia Romo, G. S., Caielli, S., Vega, B., Connolly, J., Allantaz, F., Xu, Z., . . . Pascual, V. (2011). Netting neutrophils are major inducers of type I IFN production in pediatric systemic lupus erythematosus. *Science Translational Medicine*, *2*, 73−20.

Garey, K. W., Sethi, S., Yadav, Y., & DuPont, H. L. (2008). Meta-analysis to assess risk factors for recurrent *Clostridium difficile* infection. *Journal of Hospital Infections*, *70*, 298−304. Available from https://doi.org/10.1016/j.jhin.2008.08.012.

Ginsburg, I. (2002). Role of lipoteichoic acid in infection and inflammation. *Lancet Infectious Disease*, *2*, 171−179. Available from https://doi.org/10.1016/S1473-3099(02)00226-8.

Gonzalez, D. J., Corriden, R., Akong-Moore, K., Olson, J., Dorrestein, P. C., & Nizet, V. (2014). N-terminal ArgD peptides from the classical *Staphylococcus aureus* agr system have cytotoxic and proinflammatory activities. *Chemical Biology*, *21*, 1457−1462. Available from https://doi.org/10.1016/j.chembiol.2014.09.015.

Griffin, A. J., & McSorley, S. J. (2011). Development of protective immunity to *Salmonella*, a mucosal pathogen with a systemic agenda. *Mucosal Immunology*, *4*, 371−382. Available from https://doi.org/10.1038/mi.2011.2.

Grinstein, S. (2007). Unconventional roles of the NADPH oxidase: Signaling, ion homeostasis, and cell death. *Science's STKE: Signal Transduction Knowledge Environment*, *11*, 23−34.

Guimaraes Costa, A. B., Nascimento, M. T., Froment, G. S. Soares, R. P. Morgado, F. N., ConceiçaoSilva, F., & Saraiva, E. M. (2009). *Leishmania amazonensis* promastigotes induce and are killed by neutrophil extracellular traps. *Proceedings of the National Academy of Sciences of the United States of America*, *106*, 67486753.

Halverson, T. W., Wilton, M., Poon, K. K. H., Petri, B., & Lewenza, S. (2015). DNA is an antimicrobial component of neutrophil extracellular traps. *PLOS Pathogens.*, *11*(1), e1004593.

Harada, A., Sekido, N., Akahoshi, T., Wada, T., & Mukaida, N. (1994). Essential involvement of interleukin-8 (IL-8) in acute inflammation. *Journal of Leukocyte Biology*, *56*, 559−564.

Hemmers, S., Teijaro, J. R., Arandjelovic, S., & Mowen, K. A. (2011). PAD4-mediated neutrophil extracellular trap formation is not required for immunity against influenza infection. *PLoS One*, *6*, e22043. Available from https://doi.org/10.1371/journal.pone.0022043.

Hering, N. A., Fromm, A., Kikhney, J., Lee, I. F., Moter, A., & Schulzke, J. D. (2016). *Yersinia enterocolitica* affects intestinal barrier function in the colon. *Journal of Infectious Disease*, *213*, 1157−1162. Available from https://doi.org/10.1093/infdis/jiv571.

Hoeksema, M., Tripathi, S., White, M., Qi, L., Taubenberger, J., & van Eijk, M. (2015). Arginine-rich histones have strong antiviral activity for influenza A viruses. *Innate Immunity*, *21*, 736−745. Available from https://doi.org/10.1177/1753425915593794.

Ibarra, J. A., & Steele-Mortimer, O. (2009). *Salmonella* − The ultimate insider. *Salmonella* virulence factors that modulate intracellular survival. *Cell Microbiology*, *11*, 1579−1586. Available from https://doi.org/10.1111/j.1462-5822.2009.01368.

Juneau, R. A., Pang, B., Weimer, K. E., Armbruster, C. E., & Swords, W. E. (2011). Non typeable *Haemophilus influenzae* initiates formation of neutrophil extracellular traps. *Infection and Immunity*, *79*(1), 431−438. Available from https://doi.org/10.1128/IAI.00660-10.

Kahlenberg, J. M., Carmona-Rivera, C., Smith, C. K., & Kaplan, M. J. (2013). Neutrophil extracellular trap-associated protein activation of the NLRP3 inflammasome is enhanced in lupus macrophages. *Journal of Immunology*, *190*, 1217−1226.

Kambas, K., Mitroulis, I., Apostolidou, E., Girod, A., Chrysanthopoulou, A., & Pneumatikos, I. (2012). Autophagy mediates the delivery of thrombogenic tissue factor to neutrophil extracellular traps in human sepsis. *PLoS One*, *7*, e45427. Available from https://doi.org/10.1371/journal.pone.0045427.

Kaminski, R., Chen, Y., Fischer, T., Tedaldi, E., Napoli, A., & Zhang, Y. (2016). Elimination of HIV-1 genomes from human T-lymphoid cells by CRISPR/Cas9 gene editing. *Scientific Reports*, *6*, 22555. Available from https://doi.org/10.1038/srep22555.

Kaper, J. B., Nataro, J. P., & Mobley, H. L. (2004). Pathogenic *Escherichia coli*. *Nature Reviews Microbiology*, *2*, 123−140. Available from https://doi.org/10.1038/nrmicro818.

Kaplan, M. J., & Marko, R. (2012). Neutrophil extracellular traps: Double-edged swords of innate immunity. *Journal of Immunology*, *189*(6), 2689−2695. Available from https://doi.org/10.4049/jimmunol.1201719.

Kenny, E. F., Herzig, A., Kruger, R., Muth, A., Mondal, S., Thompson, P. R., ... Zychlinsky, A. (2017). Diverse stimuli engage different neutrophil extracellular trap pathways. *Elife*, *6*. Available from https://doi.org/10.7554/eLife.24437.

Kessenbrock, K., Krumbholz, M., & Schönermarck, U. (2009). Netting neutrophils in autoimmune small-vessel vasculitis. *Nature Medicine*, *15*, 623−625.

Knight, J. S., Subramanian, V., O Dell, A. A., Yalavarthi, S., Zhao, W., Smith, C. K., ... Kaplan, M. J. (2015). Peptidylarginine deiminase inhibition disrupts NET formation and protects against kidney, skin and vascular disease in lupus-prone MRL/lpr mice. *Annals of the Rheumatic Diseases*, *74*, 2199−2206.

Knight, J. S., Zhao, W., Luo, W., Subramanian, V., O Dell, A. A., Yalavarthi, S., ... Kaplan, M. J. (2013). Peptidylarginine deiminase inhibition is immunomodulatory and vasculoprotective in murine lupus. *Journal of Clinical Investigation*, *123*, 2981−2993.

von Kökritz-Blickwede, M., Goldmann, O., Tulin, P., Heinemann, K., NorrbyTeglund, A., & Rohde, M. (2008). Phagocytosis-independent antimicrobial activity of mast cells by means of extracellular trap formation. *Blood*, *111*(6), 3070−3080. Available from https://doi.org/10.1182/blood-2007-07-104018.

Kopke, M., Straub, M., & Durre, P. (2013). *Clostridium difcile* is an autotrophic bacterial pathogen. *PLoS One*, *8*, e62157. Available from https://doi.org/10.1371/journal.pone.0062157.

Kouzarides, T. (2007). Chromatin modifications and their function. *Cell*, *128*, 693−705.

Lande, R., Ganguly, D., Facchinetti, V., Frasca, L., Conrad, C., Gregorio, J., ... Gilliet, M. (2011). Neutrophils activate plasmacytoid dendritic cells by releasing selfDNA−peptide complexes in systemic lupus erythematosus. *Science Translational Medicine*, *3*, 73ra19.

Lange, K., Buerger, M., Stallmach, A., & Bruns, T. (2016). Effects of Antibiotics on Gut Microbiota. *Digestive diseases*, *34*, 260−268.

Lee, M. J., Liu, H., Barker, B. M., Snarr, B. D., Gravelat, F. N., & Al Abdallah, Q. (2015). The fungal exopolysaccharide galactosaminogalactan mediates virulence by enhancing resistance to neutrophil extracellular traps. *PLoS Pathogens*, *11*, e1005187. Available from https://doi.org/10.1371/journal.ppat.1005187.

Lénárt, P., Rabut, G., Daigle, N., Hand, A. R., Terasaki, M., & Ellenberg, J. (2003). Nuclear envelope breakdown in starfish oocytes proceeds by partial NPC disassembly followed by a rapidly spreading fenestration of nuclear membranes. *Journal of Cell Biology*, *160*, 1055−1068.

Lewis, H. D., Liddle, J., Coote, J. E., Atkinson, S. J., Barker, M. D., Bax, B. D., ... Chen, Y. H. (2015). Inhibition of PAD4 activity is sufficient to disrupt mouse and human NET formation. *Nature Chemical Biology*, *11*, 189−191.

Li, P., Li, M., Lindberg, M. R., Kennett, M. J., Xiong, N., & Wang, Y. (2010). PAD4 is essential for antibacterial innate immunity mediated by neutrophil extracellular traps. *Journal of Experimental Medicine*, *207*, 1853−1862.

Lim, M. B. H., Kuiper, J. W. P., Katchky, A., Goldberg, H., & Glogauer, M. (2011). Rac2 is required for the formation of neutrophil extracellular traps. *Journal of Leukocyte Biology*, *90*, 771−776.

Liu, G. Y. (2009). Molecular pathogenesis of *Staphylococcus aureus* infection. *Pediatric Research*, *65*, 71R−77RR. Available from https://doi.org/10.1203/PDR.0b013e31819dc44d.

Lood, C., Blanco, L. P., Purmalek, M. M., Carmona-Rivera, C., Ravin, S. S. D., Smith, C. K., ... Kaplan, M. J. (2016). Neutrophil extracellular traps enriched in oxidized mitochondrial DNA are interferogenic and contribute to lupus-like disease. *Nature Medicine*, *22*, 146−153.

Luger, K., Mader, A. W., Richmond, R. K., Sargent, D. F., & Richmond, T. J. (2011). Crystal structure of the nucleosome core particle at 2.8 A resolution. *Nature, 389,* 251−260.

Ma, R., Li, T., Cao, M., Si, Y., Wu, X., Zhao, L., . . . Shi, J. (2016). Extracellular DNA traps released by acute promyelocytic leukemia cells through autophagy. *Cell Death and Disease, 7,* e2283.

Malachowa, N., Kobayashi, S. D., Freedman, B., Dorward, D. W., & DeLeo, F. R. (2013). Staphylococcus aureus leukotoxin GH promotes formation of neutrophil extracellular traps. *Journal of Immunology, 191,* 6022−6029.

Martyn, K. D., Kim, M. J., & Quinn, M. T. (2005). p21-Activated kinase (Pak) regulates NADPH oxidase activation in human neutrophils. *Blood, 106,* 3962−3969

Mayer, F. L., Wilson, D., & Hube, B. (2013). *Candida albicans* pathogenicity mechanisms. *Virulence, 4,* 119−128. Available from https://doi.org/10.4161/viru.22913.

McInturff, A. M., Cody, M. J., Elliott, E. A., Glenn, J. W., Rowley, J. W., Rondina, M. T., & Yost, C. C. (2012). Mammalian target of rapamycin regulates neutrophil extracellular trap formation via induction of hypoxia-inducible factor 1 α. *Blood, 120,* 3118−3125.

Metzler, K. D., Goosmann, C., Lubojemska, A., Zychlinsky, A., & Papayannopoulos, V. (2014). A myeloperoxidase-containing complex regulates neutrophil elastase release and actin dynamics during NETosis. *Cell Reports, 8,* 883−896.

Mitroulis, I., Kambas, K., Chrysanthopoulou, A., Skendros, P., Apostolidou, E., Kourtzelis, I., . . . Ritis, K. (2011). Neutrophil extracellular trap formation is associated with IL-1beta and autophagy-related signaling in gout. *PLoS One, 6,* e29318.

Mollerherm, H., Neumann, A., Schilcher, K., Blodkamp, S., Zeitouni, N. E., & Dersch, P. (2015). *Yersinia enterocolitica*-mediated degradation of neutrophil extracellular traps (NETs). *FEMS Microbiology Letters, 362,* fnv192. Available from https://doi.org/10.1093/femsle/fnv192.

Moorthy, A. N., Narasaraju, T., Rai, P., Perumalsamy, R., Tan, K. B., & Wang, S. (2013). In vivo and in vitro studies on the roles of neutrophil extracellular traps during secondary pneumococcal pneumonia afer primary pulmonary influenza infection. *Frontiers in Immunology, 4,* 56. Available from https://doi.org/10.3389/fmmu.2013.00056.

Moorthy, A. N., Rai, P., Jiao, H., Wang, S., Tan, K. B., & Qin, L. (2016). Capsules of virulent pneumococcal serotypes enhance formation of neutrophil extracellular traps during in vivo pathogenesis of pneumonia. *Oncotarget, 7,* 19327−19340. Available from https://doi.org/10.18632/oncotarget.8451.

Moreno-Altamirano, M. M., Rodriguez-Espinosa, O., Rojas-Espinosa, O., PliegoRivero, B., & Sanchez-Garcia, F. J. (2015). Dengue virus serotype-2 interferes with the formation of neutrophil extracellular traps. *Intervirology, 58,* 250−259. Available from https://doi.org/10.1159/000440723.

Mulcahy, H., Charron-Mazenod, L., & Lewenza, S. (2008). Extracellular DNA chelates cations and induces antibiotic resistance in *Pseudomonas aeruginosa* bioflms. *PLoS Pathogens, 4,* e1000213. Available from https://doi.org/10.1371/journal.ppat.1000213.

Nathan, C. (2006). Neutrophils and immunity: Challenges and opportunities. *Nature Reviews Immunology, 6,* 173−182. Available from https://doi.org/10.1038/nri1785.

Neeli, I., Dwivedi, N., Khan, S., & Radic, M. (2009). Regulation of extracellular chromatin release from neutrophils. *Journal of Innate Immunity, 1,* 194−201.

Neeli, I., Khan, S. N., & Radic, M. (2008). Histone deimination as a response to inflammatory stimuli in neutrophils. *Journal of Immunology, 180,* 1895−1902.

Neeli, I., & Radic, M. (2013). Opposition between PKC isoforms regulates histone deimination and neutrophil extracellular chromatin release. *Frontiers in Immunology, 4,* 38.

Netea, M. G., Joosten, L. A., van der Meer, J. W., Kullberg, B. J., & van de Veerdonk, F. L. (2015). Immune defence against *Candida* fungal infections. *Nature Reviews Immunology*, *15*, 630−642. Available from https://doi.org/10.1038/nri3897.

Neumann, A., Berends, E. T., Nerlich, A., Molhoek, E. M., Gallo, R. L., & Meerloo, T. (2014). The antimicrobial peptide LL-37 facilitates the formation of neutrophil extracellular traps. *Biochemical Journal*, *464*, 3−11. Available from https://doi.org/10.1042/BJ20140778.

Nusrat, A., von Eichel-Streiber, C., Turner, J. R., Verkade, P., Madara, J. L., & Parkos, C. A. (2001). *Clostridium difcile* toxins disrupt epithelial barrier function by altering membrane microdomain localization of tight junction proteins. *Infection and Immunity*, *69*, 1329−1336. Available from https://doi.org/10.1128/IAI.69.3.1329-1336.2001.

Oehmcke, S., Morgelin, M., & Herwald, H. (2009). Activation of the human contact system on neutrophil extracellular traps. *Journal of Innate Immunity*, *1*, 225−230.

Paape, M. J., Bannerman, D. D., Zhao, X., & Lee, J. W. (2003). The bovine neutrophil: Structure and function in blood and milk. *Veterinary Research*, *34*, 597−627.

Pacello, F., Ceci, P., Ammendola, S., Pasquali, P., Chiancone, E., & Battistoni, A. (2008). Periplasmic Cu, Zn superoxide dismutase and cytoplasmic Dps concur in protecting *Salmonella enterica* serovar Typhimurium from extracellular reactive oxygen species. *Biochimica et Biophysica Acta*, *1780*, 226−232. Available from https://doi.org/10.1016/j.bbagen.2007.12.001.

Papayannopoulos, V., Metzler, K. D., Hakkim, A., & Zychlinsky, A. (2010). Neutrophil elastase and myeloperoxidase regulate the formation of neutrophil extracellular traps. *Journal of Cell Biology*, *191*, 677−691.

Park, Y. J., & Luger, K. (2008). Histone chaperones in nucleosome eviction and histone exchange. *Current Opinion in Structural Biology*, *18*, 282−289.

Parker, H., Dragunow, M., Hampton, M. B., Kettle, A. J., & Winterbourn, C. C. (2012). Requirements for NADPH oxidase and myeloperoxidase in neutrophil extracellular trap formation differ depending on the stimulus. *Journal of Leukocyte Biology*, *92*, 841−849.

Pedersen, F., Marwitz, S., Holz, O., Kirsten, A., Bahmer, T., & Waschki, B. (2015). Neutrophil extracellular trap formation and extracellular DNA in sputum of stable COPD patients. *Respiratory Medicine*, *109*, 1360−1362. Available from https://doi.org/10.1016/j.rmed.2015.08.008.

Perdomo, J. J., Gounon, P., & Sansonetti, P. J. (1994). Polymorphonuclear leukocyte transmigration promotes invasion of colonic epithelial monolayer by *Shigella flexneri*. *Journal of Clinical Investigation*, *93*, 633−643. Available from https://doi.org/10.1172/JCI117011.

Persson, Y. A., Blomgran-Julinder, R., Rahman, S., Zheng, L., & Stendahl, O. (2008). *Mycobacterium tuberculosis*-induced apoptotic neutrophils trigger a proinflammatory response in macrophages through release of heat shock protein 72, acting in synergy with the bacteria. *Microbes and Infection*, *10*, 233−240. Available from https://doi.org/10.1016/j.micinf.2007.11.007.

Phalipon, A., & Sansonetti, P. J. (2007). Shigellas ways of manipulating the host intestinal innate and adaptive immune system: A tool box for survival? *Immunology and Cell Biology*, *85*, 119−129. Available from https://doi.org/10.1038/sj.icb7100025.

Pieterse, E., Rother, N., Yanginlar, C., Hilbrands, L. B., & van der Vlag, J. (2016). Neutrophils discriminate between lipopolysaccharides of different bacterial sources and selectively release neutrophil extracellular traps. *Frontiers in Immunology*, *7*, 484. Available from https://doi.org/10.3389/fmmu.2016.00484.

Pilsczek, F. H., Salina, D., Poon, K. K., Fahey, C., Yipp, B. G., & Sibley, C. D. (2010). A novel mechanism of rapid nuclear neutrophil extracellular trap formation in response to *Staphylococcus aureus*. *Journal of Immunology*, *185*, 7413−7425. Available from https://doi.org/10.4049/jimmunol.1000675.

Pilsczek, F. H., Salina, D., Poon, K. K., Fahey, C., Yipp, B. G., & Sibley, C. D. (2015). A novel mechanism of rapid nuclear neutrophil extracellular trap formation in response to *Staphylococcus aureus*. *Journal of Immunology*, *185*, 7413−7425. Available from https://doi.org/10.4049/jimmunol.1000675.

Price, M. O., Atkinson, S. J., & Knaus, U. G. (2002). Rac activation induces NADPH oxidase activity in transgenic COSphox cells, and the level of superoxide production is exchange factor-dependent. *The Journal of Biological Chemistry*, *277*, 19220−19228.

Qiu, S. L., Zhang, H., Tang, Q. Y., Bai, J., He, Z. Y., Zhang, J. Q., ... Zhong, X. N. (2017). Neutrophil extracellular traps induced by cigarette smoke activate plasmacytoid dendritic cells. *Thorax*, *72*, 1084−1093,

Raad, H., Paclet, M. H., Boussetta, T., Kroviarski, Y., Morel, F., Quinn, M. T., ... El-Benna, J. (2009). Regulation of the phagocyte NADPH oxidase activity: phosphorylation of gp91phox/NOX2 by protein kinase C enhances its diaphorase activity and binding to Rac2, p67phox, and p47phox. *FASEB Journal*, *23*, 1011−1022.

Ramos-Kichik, V., Mondragon-Flores, R., Mondragon-Castelan, M., GonzalezPozos, S., Muniz-Hernandez, S., & Rojas-Espinosa, O. (2009). Neutrophil extracellular traps are induced by *Mycobacterium tuberculosis*. *Tuberculosis*, *89*, 29−37. Available from https://doi.org/10.1016/j.tube.2008.09.00.

Reidl, J., & Klose, K. E. (2002). *Vibrio cholerae* and cholera: Out of the water and into the host. *FEMS Microbiology Reviews*, *26*, 125−139. Available from https://doi.org/10.1111/j.1574-6976.2002.tb00605.

Remijsen, Q., Berghe, T. V., & Wirawan, E. (2011). Neutrophil extracellular trap cell death requires both autophagy and superoxide generation. *Cell Research*, *21*, 290−304.

Rocha, J. D., Nascimento, M. T., Decote-Ricardo, D., Corte-Real, S., Morrot, A., & Heise, N. (2015). Capsular polysaccharides from *Cryptococcus neoformans* modulate production of neutrophil extracellular traps (NETs) by human neutrophils. *Scientific Reports*, *5*, 8008. Available from https://doi.org/10.1038/srep08008.

Rodriguez-Espinosa, O., Rojas-Espinosa, O., Moreno-Altamirano, M. M., LopezVillegas, E. O., & Sanchez-Garcia, F. J. (2015). Metabolic requirements for neutrophil extracellular traps formation. *Immunology*, *145*, 213−224. Available from https://doi.org/10.1111/imm.1243.

Rohm, M., Grimm, M. J., DAuria, A. C., Almyroudis, N. G., Segal, B. H., & Urban, C. F. (2014). NADPH oxidase promotes neutrophil extracellular trap formation in pulmonary aspergillosis. *Infection and Immunity*, *82*, 1766−1777. Available from https://doi.org/10.1128/IAI.00096-14.

Saitoh, T., Komano, J., Saitoh, Y., Misawa, T., Takahama, M., Kozaki, T., ... Akira, S. (2012). Neutrophil extracellular traps mediate a host defense response to human immunodeficiency virus-1. *Cell Host & Microbe*, *12*, 109−116. Available from https://doi.org/10.1016/j.chom.2012.05.015.

Seeley, E. J., Matthay, M. A., & Wolters, P. J. (2012). Inflection points in sepsis biology: From local defense to systemic organ injury. *American Journal of Physiology Lung Cellular and Molecular Physiology*, *303*, L355−L363. Available from https://doi.org/10.1152/ajplung.00069.2012.

Segal, B. H., & Romani, L. R. (2009). Invasive aspergillosis in chronic granulomatous disease. *Medical Mycology*, *47*, S282−S290. Available from https://doi.org/10.1080/13693780902736620.

Seper, A., Hosseinzadeh, A., Gorkiewicz, G., Lichtenegger, S., Roier, S., & Leitner, D. R. (2013). *Vibrio cholerae* evades neutrophil extracellular traps by the activity of two extracellular nucleases. *PLoS Pathogen*, *9*, e1003614. Available from https://doi.org/10.1371/journal.ppat.1003614.

Sollberger, G., Amulic, B., & Zychlinsky, A. (2016). Neutrophil extracellular trap formation is independent of de novo gene expression. *PLoS One*, *11*, e0157454.

Sollberger, G., Choidas, A., Burn, G. L., Habenberger, P., Di Lucrezia, R., Kordes, S., ... Zychlinsky, A. (2018). Gasdermin D plays a vital role in the generation of neutrophil extracellular traps*Science Immunology*, *3*, pii: eaar6689. Available from https://doi.org/10.1126/sciimmunol.aar6689.

Sorg, J. A., & Sonenshein, A. L. (2010). Inhibiting the initiation of *Clostridium difficile* spore germination using analogs of chenodeoxycholic acid, a bile acid. *Journal of Bacteriology*, *192*, 4983−4990. Available from https://doi.org/10.1128/JB.00610-10.

Sousa-Rocha, D., Thomaz-Tobias, M., Diniz, L. F., Souza, P. S., Pinge-Filho, P., & Toledo, K. A. (2015). *Trypanosoma cruzi* and its soluble antigens induce NET release by stimulating Toll-like receptors. *PLoS One*, *10*, e0139569.

Spinner, J. L., Seo, K. S., OLoughlin, J. L., Cundiff, J. A., Minnich, S. A., & Bohach, G. A. (2010). Neutrophils are resistant to Yersinia YopJ/P-induced apoptosis and are protected from ROS-mediated cell death by the type III secretion system. *PLoS One*, *5*, e9279. Available from https://doi.org/10.1371/journal.pone.0009279.

Steinberg, B. E., & Grinstein, S. (2007). Unconventional roles of the NADPH oxidase: Signaling, ion homeostasis, and cell death. *Science STKE*, *379*, pe11.

Talbert, P. B., & Henikoff, S. (2010). Histone variants—Ancient wrap artists of the epigenome. *Nature Review of Molecular Cell Biology*, *11*, 264−275.

Tammavongsa, V., Missiakas, D. M., & Schneewind, O. (2014). *Staphylococcus aureus* degrades neutrophil extracellular traps to promote immune cell death. *Science*, *342*, 863−866. Available from https://doi.org/10.1126/science.1242255.

Tanaka, K., Koike, Y., Shimura, T., Okigami, M., Ide, S., & Toiyama, Y. (2014). In vivo characterization of neutrophil extracellular traps in various organs of a murine sepsis model. *PLoS One*, *9*, e111888. Available from https://doi.org/10.1371/journal.pone.0111888.

Tang, S., Zhang, Y., Yin, S. W., Gao, X. J., Shi, W. W., Wang, Y., ... Zhang, J. B. (2015). Neutrophil extracellular trap formation is associated with autophagy-related signalling in ANCA-associated vasculitis. *Clinical and experimental immunology*, *180*, 408−418.

Tobias, A. F., Ulrike, A., Christian, G., Robert, H., Ilka, S., & Volker, W. (2007). Novel cell death program leads to neutrophil extracellular traps. *Journal of Cell Biology*, *176*(2), 231−241. Available from https://doi.org/10.1083/jcb.200606027.

Tripathi, S., Verma, A., Kim, E. J., White, M. R., & Hartshorn, K. L. (2014). LL-37 modulates human neutrophil responses to influenza A virus. *Journal of Leukocyte Biology*, *96*, 931−938. Available from https://doi.org/10.1189/jlb.4A1113-604RR.

Troeger, A., & Williams, D. A. (2013). Hematopoietic-specific Rho GTPases Rac2 and RhoH and human blood disorders. *Experimental Cell Research*, *319*, 2375−2383.

Urban, C. F., Ermert, D., Schmid, M., Abu-Abed, U., Goosmann, C., Nacken, W., ... Zychlinsky, A. (2009). Neutrophil extracellular traps contain calprotectin, a cytosolic protein complex involved in host defense against *Candida albicans. PLoS Pathogens*, *5*, e1000639.

Urban, C. F., Reichard, U., Brinkmann, V., & Zychlinsky, A. (2006). Neutrophil extracellular traps capture and kill *Candida albicans* yeast and hyphal forms. *Cellular Microbiology*, *8*(4), 668−676. Available from https://doi.org/10.1111/j.1462-5822.2005.00659.

Van Dervort, A. L., Yan, L., Madara, P. J., Cobb, J. P., & Wesley, R. A. (1994). Nitric oxide regulates endotoxin-induced TNF-alpha production by human neutrophils. *Journal of Immunology*, *152*, 4102−4109.

Vorobjeva, N. V. (2013). NADPH oxidase of neutrophils and diseases associated with its dysfunction. *Immunologiya*, *34*, 232−238.

Waisberg, M., Molina-Cruz, A., Mizurini, D. M., Gera, N., Sousa, B. C., & Ma, D. (2014). *Plasmodium falciparum* infection induces expression of a mosquito salivary protein (Agaphelin) that targets neutrophil function and inhibits thrombosis without impairing hemostasis. *PLoS Pathogens*, *10*, e1004338. Available from https://doi.org/10.1371/journal. ppat.100433.

Wang, Y., Li, M., Stadler, S., Correll, S., Li, P., Wang, D., ... Coonrod, S. A. (2009). Histone hypercitrullination mediates chromatin decondensation and neutrophil extracellular trap formation. *Journal of Cell Biology*, *184*, 205−213.

Wartha, F., Beiter, K., Albiger, B., Fernebro, J., Zychlinsky, A., & Normark, S. (2007). Capsule and D-alanylated lipoteichoic acids protect *Streptococcus pneumoniae* against neutrophil extracellular traps. *Cellular Microbiology*, *9*(5), 1162−1171. Available from https://doi.org/10.1111/j.1462-5822.2006.00857.x.

Wildhagen, K. C., Garcia de Frutos, P., Reutelingsperger, C. P., Schrijver, R., Areste, C., Ortega-Gomez, A., ... Nicolaes, G. A. (2014). Nonanticoagulant heparin prevents histone-mediated cytotoxicity in vitro and improves survival in sepsis. *Blood*, *123*, 1098−1101.

Wu, F., Tyml, K., & Wilson, J. X. (2008). iNOS expression requires NADPH oxidasedependent redox signaling in microvascular endothelial cells. *Journal of Cellular Physiology*, *217*, 207−214.

Xu, J., Zhang, X., Pelayo, R., Monestier, M., Ammollo, C. T., Semeraro, F., ... Esmon, C. T. (2009). Extracellular histones are major mediators of death in sepsis. *Nature Medicine*, *15*, 1318−1321.

Yang, H., & Biermann, M. H. (2016). New insights into Neutrophil extracellular Traps: Mechanisms of Formation and Role in inflammation. *Frontiers in immunology*, *7*, 1−8. Available from https://doi.org/10.3389/fimmu.2016.00302.

Young, R. L., Malcolm, K. C., Kret, J. E., Caceres, S. M., Poch, K. R., & Nichols, D. P. (2011). Neutrophil extracellular trap (NET)-mediated killing of *Pseudomonas aeruginosa*: Evidence of acquired resistance within the CF airway, independent of CFTR. *PLoS One*, *6*, e23637. Available from https://doi.org/10.1371/journal.pone.0023637.

Yousefi, S., Mihalache, C., Kozlowski, E., Schmid, I., & Simon, H. U. (2009). Viable neutrophils release mitochondrial DNA to form neutrophil extracellular traps. *Cell Death and Differentiation*, *16*(11), 1438−1444.

Zhu, L., Kuang, Z., Wilson, B. A., & Lau, G. W. (2013). Competence-independent activity of pneumococcal EndA [corrected] mediates degradation of extracellular DNA and nets and is important for virulence. *PLoS One*, *8*, e70363. Available from https://doi.org/10.1371/journal.pone.0070363.

Zigra, P. I., Maipa, V. E., & Alamanos, Y. P. (2007). Probiotics and remission of ulcerative colitis: A systematic review. *Netherlands Journal of Medicine*, *65*, 411−418.

Further reading

Brinkmann, V., Laube, B., Abu, Abed, U., Goosmann, C., & Zychlinsky, A. (2010). Neutrophil extracellular traps: How to generate and visualize them. *Journal of Visualized Experiments*, *36*, 1724.

Gavillet, M., Martinod, K., Renella, R., Wagner, D. D., & Williams, D. A. (2017). A key role for Rac and Pak signaling in neutrophil extracellular traps (NETs) formation defines a new potential therapeutic target. *American Journal of Hematology*, *93*(2), 269−276. Available from https://doi.org/10.1002/ajh.24970.

Palmer, L. J., Cooper, P. R., Ling, M. R., Wright, H. J., Huissoon, A., & Chapple, I. L. (2012). Hypochlorous acid regulates neutrophil extracellular trap release in humans. *Clinical and Experimental Immunology, 167*, 261−268.

Patel, S., Kumar, S., & Jyoti, A. (2010). Nitric oxide donors release extracellular traps from human neutrophils by augmenting free radical generation. *Nitric Oxide, 22*(3), 226−234.

Roberts, H. (2016). Characterization of neutrophil function in Papillon-Lefevre syndrome. *Journal of Leukocyte Biology, 100*, 433−444.

Saskia, H., John, R. T., Sanja, A., & Kerra, A. M. (2011). PAD4-mediated neutrophil extracellular trap formation is not required for immunity against influenza infection. *PLoS One, 6*(7), e22043. Available from https://doi.org/10.1371/journal.pone.0022043.

Sorensen, O. E., et al. (2014). Papillon-Lefevre syndrome patient reveals species-dependent requirements for neutrophil defenses. *Journal of Clinical Investigation, 124*, 4539−4548.

Spaan, A. N., Surewaard, B. G., Nijland, R., & van Strijp, J. A. (2013). Neutrophils vs *Staphylococcus aureus*: A biological tug of war. *Annual Review of Microbiology, 67*, 629−650.

Walker, M. J., et al. (2007). DNase Sda1 provides selection pressure for a switch to invasive group A streptococcal infection. *Nature Medicine, 13*, 981−985.

Yoo, D. G., et al. (2014). Release of cystic fibrosis airway inflammatory markers from *Pseudomonas aeruginosa*-stimulated human neutrophils involves NADPH oxidase-dependent extracellular DNA trap formation. *Journal of Immunology, 192*, 4728−4738.

Yousefi, S., Gold, J. A., & Andina, N. (2008). Catapult-like release of mitochondrial DNA by eosinophils contributes to antibacterial defense. *Nature Medicine, 14*(9), 949−953.

Chapter 3

Factors regulating NETosis

Autophagy, apoptosis, and necrosis are three different forms of cell death which is a vital biological process imperative for regulation of physiological growth and development. These biological processes exhibit unique morphological features and activate specific signaling pathways. The final cell fate is a consequence of cross talk between these distinct signaling pathways that interconnect or even overlap (Chen, Kang, & Fu, 2018). These processes have been studied in conjunction with NETosis and there are reports on the involvement of these cell death pathways in the process of NETosis.

Autophagy in NETosis

Autophagy is a key mechanism for cell endurance and maintenance of homeostasis. It is a self-digesting process that helps in clearance of damaged organelles and misfolded proteins during cellular stress along with recycling of organelles and cytosolic macromolecules for essential nutrient supply by targeting intracellular cargo for degradation in endosomes and lysosomes (Klionsky & Emr, 2000). This is morphologically characterized by accumulation of autophagic vacuoles. Serious defects in autophagy are therefore considered lethal. Additionally, autophagy also contributes to lymphocyte development and survival, antigen presentation and T-cell proliferation.

Autophagy has been found to be involved in the mechanism of phorbol myristate acetate (PMA)−induced neutrophil extracellular traps (NETs) formation and promoted this process (Remijsen, Vanden Berghe, et al., 2011). Autophagy also plays a positive role in the process of formyl-methionyl-leucyl-phenylalanine (fMLP)−induced or interleukin (IL)-1β−induced NETs formation (Itakura & McCarty, 2013; Mitroulis, 2011), however, negatively regulates the NETs formation induced by lipopolysaccharide (LPS) (McInturff et al., 2012). Even if autophagy is inhibited there is no effect on NOX2 activity induced by PMA. For NET formation, intracellular chromatin decondensation is essential, which can be achieved by either inhibiting the process of autophagy or NOX2 (Remijsen, Kuijpers et al., 2011). Therefore it seems that depending on the stimulants for neutrophils the role of autophagy in NETs formation varies.

NETosis. DOI: https://doi.org/10.1016/B978-0-12-816147-0.00003-4

Various autophagic stimulants induce NETosis

Antineutrophil cytoplasmic antibodies

Autophagy vacuolization has been detected in neutrophils treated with myeloperoxidase (MPO)- and proteinase 3 (PR3)-ANCA-positive immunoglobulin (IgG) and is speculated that autophagy could facilitate the release of ANCA-positive-IgG induced NETs (Sha et al., 2016). It has also been reported that inhibiting the autophagy has inhibited the NET formation (Remijsen, Kuijpers et al., 2011; Remijsen, Vanden Berghe et al., 2011). In 2016 Sha et al. provided evidence for induction of autophagy by MPO- and PR3-ANCA-positive IgG. NETs formation is inhibited when autophagy is blocked. Dysregulated NETs formation contributes to the pathogenesis of ANCA-associated vasculitis (AAV). ANCA-induced NETs formation triggers vasculitis and facilitates the autoimmune response against neutrophil constituents in AAV patients (Kessenbrock, Krumbholz, & Schönermarck, 2009). ANCAs, the serological markers of AAV, are specific for the cytoplasmic constituents of neutrophils, particularly, PR3 and MPO. ANCA-IgG, which is specific for MPO and PR3, could induce primed human neutrophils to form NETs in vitro.

Phorbol myristate acetate

PMA enhances cell autophagy induced by rapamycin and also acts as an activator of extracellular signal−regulated kinase (ERK) signal pathway (Ying, 2017). Autophagy was involved in the mechanism of NETs formation treated with PMA and promoted this process. Autophagy and superoxide production occur independent of each other and are involved in PMA-induced NETosis. Intracellular chromatin decondensation and NET formation following autophagy has been reported (Remijsen, Kuijpers et al., 2011; Remijsen, Vanden Berghe et al., 2011).

Bacteria-derived formyl-methionyl-leucyl-phenylalanine

Autophagy promotes NETs formation induced by the bacteria-derived peptide fMLP (Itakura & McCarty, 2013), the same as NETs formation stimulated with PMA or IL-1β (Mitroulis et al., 2011).

Mammalian target of rapamycin (mTOR) kinase plays an important role in autophagy in neutrophils by regulating the autophagic activity. After stimulation of neutrophil with fMLP and the mTOR pathway inhibition, the rate of NET release increases resulting in the formation of autophagosome. Hence fMLP-induced neutrophil autophagy is regulated by mTOR pathway. In response to fMLP rapamycin enables the NET release by the control of autophagy influx. On the contrary mTOR pathway negatively regulates NETosis downstream of formyl-peptide receptors (FPR) signaling (Itakura & McCarty, 2013). Activation of NADPH oxidase (NOX) (Sheppard et al., 2005) and the mTOR pathway (Liu et al., 2010) are regulated by the binding of fMLP to FPRs.

Lipopolysaccharide

Autophagy negatively regulates NETosis when induced with LPS (McInturff et al., 2012). The formation of osteoclasts is increased by the induction of autophagy with the LPS. LPS-induced autophagy was established when formation of autophagosome was detected by immunoblotting cell lysates with an antibody against microtubule-associated protein light chain 3 (LC3) and also by the formation of acidic vesicular organelles (AVOs, which include autolysosomes) by flow cytometry using the pH-sensitive fluorescent dye, acridine orange (Itakura & McCarty, 2013).

A summary of various autophagic inducers of NET has been provided in the Fig. 3.1.

Autophagy-related molecules in NETosis

The pathways promoting NETosis upstream of ROS are not completely understood. A number of ROS-inducing receptors (BOX 1) and kinases, such as extracellular signal−regulated kinase (ERK), microtubule-associated protein kinase (MAPK), MAPK/ERK kinase (MEK), IL-1 receptor−associated kinase (IRAK), protein kinase C (PKC), Phosphoinositide 3-kinase (PI3K), and AKT, have been linked to NETosis (DeSouza-Vieira et al., 2016). PI3K implicated in NETosis has a role in autophagy too. The lack of autophagy-associated protein, ATG7 in pro-myelocytes causes a moderate decrease in release of NET (Ma et al., 2016). mTOR involved in regulation of NETosis suppresses autophagy process (McInturff et al., 2012). However, LC3B$^+$ vacuoles that are similar to autophagosomes have been found to undergo NETosis (Tang et al., 2015).

PMA-induced chromatin decondensation requires NOX2 activity in NETosis

It has been found that along with disintegration of nuclear envelope and most granule membranes, NOX2-mediated oxidative burst (Babior, 1999) also play an important role in activation of NETosis. In due course these result in massive vacuolization (Fuchs et al., 2007), intracellular decondensation of nuclear chromatin (Wang et al., 2009) and consequently in the formation of NETs (Brinkmann et al., 2004). NOX2 is a highly regulated membrane-associated multiprotein complex and produces considerable amounts of superoxide that causes oxidative burst, hence, recognized as a controller of NETosis (Babior, 1999). PMA-induced NETosis can be inhibited by suppressing the activity of NOX2 by diphenyleneiodonium (DPI) or by eliminating it.

NOX2 when activated by PMA induces superoxide generation. Generation of reactive oxygen species (ROS) is significant because this

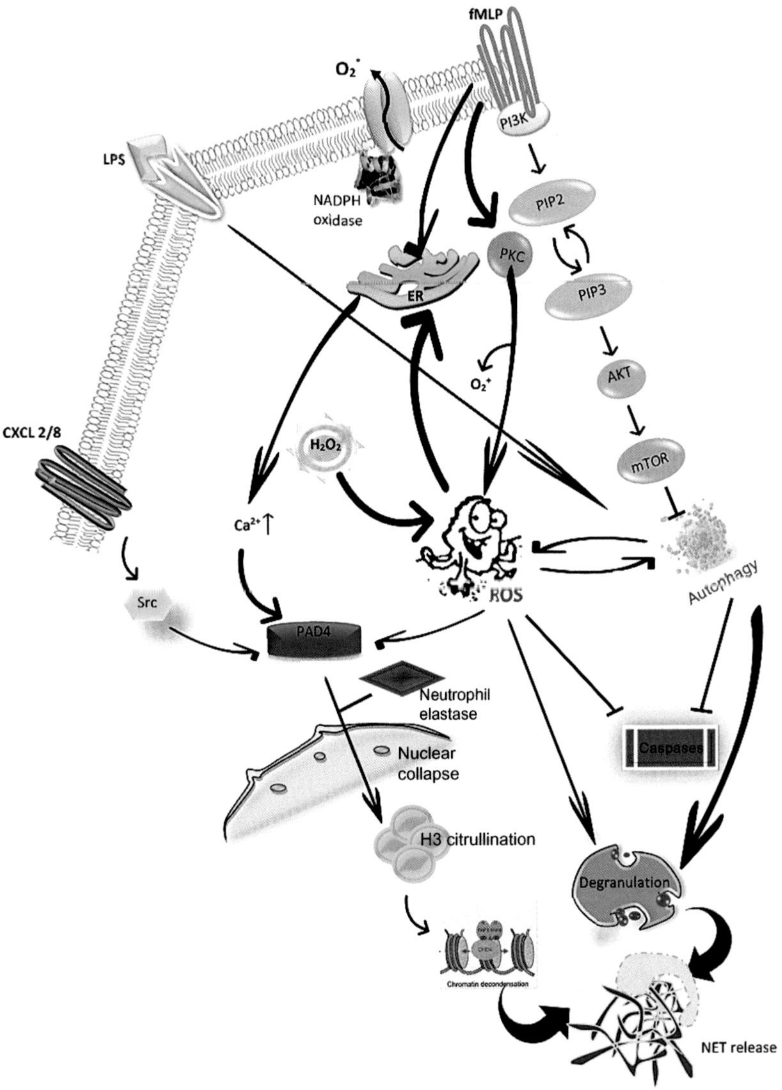

FIGURE 3.1 Autophagic inducers of NET. Lipopolysaccharide (LPS) triggers autophagy in neutrophils and sensitizes them for oxidative burst induced by NADPH oxidase. Formyl-methionyl-leucyl-phenylalanine (fMLP) induces autophagy by mammalian target of rapamycin (mTOR) pathway and increases ROS production leading to histone 3 citrullination by PAD4 and neutrophil elastase. It also induces signaling through Akt/PI3K. PI3K/Akt mTOR cascade inhibits autophagy, preventing the formation of NET. ROS along with autophagy causes chromatin decondensation and collapse of the nuclear membrane leading to NETosis, but inhibits caspase activity.

happens to be obligatory for NET induction. Even in absence of NOX2 either due to a genetic defect in its subunits or inhibition of its activity by DPI, PMA will induce cell death but with delayed kinetics as compared to uninduced normal neutrophils. Unstimulated neutrophils from chronic granulomatous disease (CGD) patients or healthy volunteers, whether or not pretreated with DPI, die spontaneously from apoptosis (Remijsen et al., 2009), but more slowly than in PMA-induced NETosis. At the time of initiation of NETosis a massive vacuolization occurs. Vacuoles were thought to emerge from the nuclear envelope and to promote its collapse before NET formation as they are produced before disintegration of the nuclear envelope. Like normal neutrophils, upon stimulation of CGD neutrophils with PMA, they undergo massive vacuolization and lose their mitochondrial potential quickly. In CGD neutrophils, during the time interval in between PMA stimulation and plasma membrane disintegration intracellular chromatin decondensation was not observed. This massive vacuolization during NETosis advocates that endoplasmic reticulum (ER) membranes might be assembled as a source of membranes along with formation of autophagosomes. If so, then a decrease in perinuclear ER membranes can lower nuclear collapse. When CGD neutrophils are induced with PMA, massive vacuolization occurs without disintegration of nuclear membrane, which defies the relationship between the disintegration of the nuclear envelope and subsequent chromatin decondensation as well as the process vacuolization (Brinkmann & Zychlinsky, 2007; Fuchs et al., 2007). This implies that some other mechanisms besides nuclear envelope disintegration are involved in the formation of vesicles and vacuoles with double membranes.

Through a process referred as priming the activity of NOX2 is sensitized by both LPS and IL-8, however, they cannot induce Nox2 activity directly (Sheppard et al., 2005), as evidenced by the inability of CGD neutrophils to undergo NETosis it is apparent that Nox2 activity is essential for NETosis (Fuchs et al., 2007). It has been further documented by Bianchi et al., 2009 that the inability of neutrophils from CGD patients to undergo NETosis correlates with their sensitivity to infection (Bianchi et al., 2009). NETosis is characterized by decondensation of intracellular chromatin and disintegration of the nuclear envelope. It has been demonstrated that Nox2 activity is required for chromatin decondensation, in intact neutrophils, the activity of NOX2 is needed for decondensation of chromatin (Yousefi & Simon, 2009).

Effect of autophagy inhibition on NETosis

Wortmannin is a cell permeable, fungal steroid metabolite acts as a potent and irreversible inhibitor of PI3Ks (Arcaro & Wymann, 1993). Autophagy is modulated by mTOR kinase and indirectly by PI3K/AKT survival pathway. In autophagy cellular materials are sequestered and delivered to the lysosome for degradation. Inhibition of PI3K with wortmannin can inhibit autophagic sequestration (Blommaart, Krause, Schellens, Vreeling-Sindelárová, & Meijer, 1997). On the other side, autophagy inhibited by wortmannin does not affect the generation of superoxide but prevents the induction of vacuolization. Hence, this inhibition without disturbing NOX2 activity prevents the intracellular chromatin decondensation which infers that during NET formation NOX2 activity is essential but not enough for the intracellular chromatin decondensation (Remijsen, Kuijpers et al., 2011; Remijsen, Vanden Berghe et al., 2011). CGD neutrophils undergoing autophagy are deficient in activity of NOX2 and therefore cannot induce intracellular chromatin decondensation. When neutrophil autophagy was inhibited intracellular chromatin decondensation was seen to be impaired, however, the neutrophils continued to undergo cell death showing characteristic features of apoptosis. Thus rather than for cell death process, autophagy is indispensable requisite in the initial stage of NETosis

Role of Toll-like receptors in autophagy

TLRs and nucleotide binding and oligomerization domain (NOD)-like receptors (NLR) are the pattern recognition receptors (PRR) which show induction of autophagy in macrophages. In response to TLR ligands neutrophils can also induce autophagy. Neutrophil autophagy can be induced by either of the two ways, i.e., phagocytosis-dependent or phagocytosis independent manner.

In elimination of intracellular microbes, TLR7 ligands stimulated autophagy plays an important role, even when the target pathogen was normally not associated with TLR7 signaling. This serves as an evidence for connecting TLR signaling and autophagy: two innate immunity defence systems, providing a possible molecular mechanism for induction of autophagy in response to pathogen invasion.

Involvement of autophagy in neutrophil extracellular trap formation during fungal infection

Autophagy plays an important role in inducing NET release in response to *Candida albicans*. *C. albicans* hyphae and live yeast both induce autophagy-mediated NETs release although distinct kinetics and mechanisms of NET induction are employed. NET formation in response to hyphal form involves autophagy but not ROS whereas NET formation triggered by *C. albicans* yeast involves both the mechanisms.

Apoptosis in NETosis

Apoptosis is a cell death mechanism mediated by caspases and involves condensation of nucleus and cytoplasm. It plays a significant role in developmental processes as this is involved in removal of interdigital cells, nonfunctional nerve cells, and activated lymphocytes (Nagata, 2018). However, it may not be involved in clearing senescent cells (red blood cells and intestinal enterocytes). Specific sets of caspases acting in cascades mediate apoptosis (deCathelineau & Henson, 2003). Apoptotic cells themselves are engulfed by macrophages hence it is hard to locate any free apoptotic cells in vivo, even in tissues where huge numbers of cells undergo apoptosis (Surh & Sprent, 1994). Thus apoptosis involves mechanisms not only for killing cells but also for recruiting macrophages (find me) and presenting a signal(s) (eat me) to the macrophages for cell engulfment (Medina & Ravichandran, 2016; Nagata et al., 2011). Although NETosis is a distinct form of cell death entirely independent from apoptosis, an alternative form of neutrophil death "ApoNETosis" reported recently has been described to be concomitant with apoptosis and NETosis (Azzouz, Khan, Sweezey, & Palaniyar, 2018). ApoNETosis, apoptosis, NETosis, have similarities as well as unique differences. Identifying the molecular steps involved in the regulation of ApoNETosis could be key to understanding certain pathobiological situations.

In intrinsic apoptosis once cytochrome c binds the adapter protein, Apaf-1, in the cytoplasm the complex forms caspase 9 by activating pro-caspase-9. Consequently, caspase 9 activates caspase-3/7 which are the effector proteins, leading to activation of caspase-activated DNase (CAD) (Simon, Yehia, & Schaffer, 2000). Fas ligand and tumor necrosis factor α (TNFα) induce extrinsic apoptosis by activating Fas and tumor necrosis factor receptor-1 (TNFR-1), respectively, which are membrane proteins (Croker et al., 2011). Death-inducing signaling complex (DISC) composed of Fas, Fas-associated protein with Death Domain (FADD), and pro-caspase-8, formation is a consequence of activation of either membrane proteins which ultimately cause activation of caspase 8 leading to the activation of effector caspases 3/7 and consequently CAD8. Depending on the phosphorylation state, caspase 8 prolongs neutrophils endurance. Members of Bcl-2 family, Bax and Bak, play an important role in neutrophil apoptosis (Jia, Parodo, Kapus, Rotstein, & Marshall, 2008). Neutrophils have elevated expressions of pro-apoptotic Bcl-2 family members, Bax and Bak, which may have some role in their observed short life spans. Pro-apoptotic Bid, Bim, and Bad are also expressed in neutrophils. Neutrophils express Mcl-1, Bcl-xl, and A1 which are antiapoptotic Bcl-2 family members (Simon, 2003).

There are many factors and signaling pathways that affect neutrophil apoptosis. On one hand, neutrophil survival is enhanced by granulocyte/macrophage colony-stimulating factor (GM-CSF), granulocyte colony-stimulating factor (G-CSF), and adenosine triphosphate (ATP), on the other hand, their apoptosis is increased by activation of certain TNF/nerve growth factor receptor family members. Although NETosis and apoptosis are conventionally two separate processes, but in terms of interaction between apoptosis and NETosis, caspase activity (a hallmark of apoptosis) was found to be missing during induction of NETosis (Simon, 2003).

ApoNETosis

Similar to apoptosis and all types of NETosis, apoNETosis requires increased ROS production, specifically of mitochondrial origin. Ultraviolet (UV) at high doses can induce apoptosis and Netosis in the same neutrophil. During UV-induced ApoNETosis, NOX is inactive signifying that the process is NOX-independent, however, MAPK p38 activation is required. ApoNETosis similar to other forms of NOX-independent NETosis, requires transcriptional activation (Azzouz et al., 2018). However, histones are not citrullinated during this process, marking it different from other forms of NOX-independent NETosis. This indicates that during UV exposure of neutrophils, there is no change in intracellular calcium concentration and peptidyl arginine deiminase 4 (PAD4) activation. In addition, there is cleavage of caspase-3 suggestive of the activation of apoptotic pathways, like other types of apoptosis. However, similar to other forms of NOX-independent NETosis, there is increased transcriptional firing during ApoNETosis (Fig. 3.2).

Molecules at the interface of apoptosis and NETosis

Hypertonic sodium chloride (NaCl) encourages apoptosis at the same time suppressing NOX2-dependent NETosis. Quite the reverse NOX2-independent NETosis is not suppressed by hypertonic solutions. Ionomycin-induced NETosis is suppressed by hypertonic saline but enhances A23187-induced NETosis, however, no change in *Staphylococcus aureus*−induced NETosis occurs. This also suppresses NOX2-dependent NETosis induced by several agonists; on the other hand, it has number of outcomes on neutrophil death induced by NOX2-independent NETosis agonists. The increasing concentrations of mannitol and D-sorbitol, nonionic osmolytes suppresses ROS production and PMA-, LPS-, and ionomycin-mediated NETosis. Hypertonic saline suppresses NETosis and promotes apoptosis as an alternate pathway of programmed cell death is revealed by cleaved caspase-3 (cCasp-3) which is an apoptotic marker (Nadesalingam, Chen, Farahvash, & Khan, 2018).

Olfactomedin 4 (OLFM4) is present in roughly 20%−25% of neutrophils which is a specific granule protein. Its presence is not regulated at the level of transcription (Clemmensen et al., 2012). In in vivo OLFM4-positive and OLFM4-negative neutrophil subpopulations are recruited equally to the inflammatory sites and similarly undergo apoptosis and also phagocytose bacteria. Upon in vivo transmigration, only limited OLFM4 was released, whereas in vitro degranulation required strong secretagogues, namely cytochalasin B and ionomycin. However, in response to PMA, OLFM4 was released upon NETs formation and was found in only a fraction of the NETs (Welin et al., 2013).

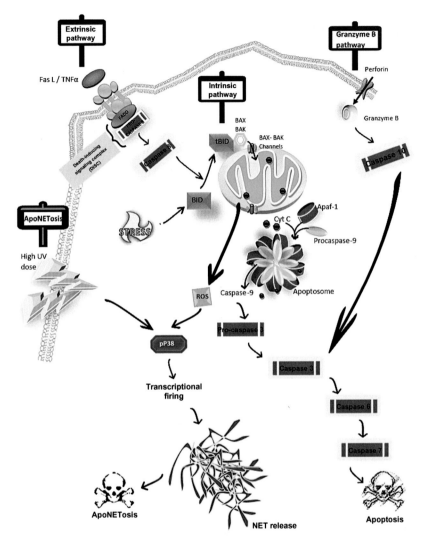

FIGURE 3.2 ApoNETosis versus apoptosis (extrinsic, intrinsic, and granzyme B) pathways. FasL or TNFα binds to the transmembrane death receptor, Fas-associated protein with death domain (FADD) which recruits pro-caspase-8 molecules forming a death-inducing signaling complex (DISC) with caspase-8. Eventually this activates caspases 3 and 7 by proteolytic processing which further activates caspase cascade leading to the death. In some conditions, cross talk between extrinsic and intrinsic pathways occurs. Certain stimuli-like cell stress can activate BH3 only protein BID. Caspase-8 proteolyze BID and form truncated BID (tBID). Activation of BID promotes assembly of BAK-BAX oligomer on the outer membrane of mitochondria. BAX-BAK allows efflux of Cytochrome c into cytosol. Cytochrome C assembles with Apaf-1 and pro-caspase-9 forms active caspase-9 which also participates in further caspase activation events leading to cell death. Granzyme also triggers apoptosis of target cells. This is a family of structurally related serine proteases stored within the cytotoxic granules of cytotoxic lymphocyte which are delivered by perforin. Perforin forms a pore and targets the cell to allow the entry of granzymes, which is similar to caspase in terms of activity. Granzyme cleaves its substrate and mediate the effector caspase-3 and initiator caspase-8 to regulate the apoptosis pathway. UV-induced ApoNETosis is a result of MAPK p38 activation and increased ROS production which is mitochondrial in origin leading to transcriptional firing.

Phagocytotic uptake: Apotosis versus NETosis

Phagocytotic removal of NETs and neutrophils undergoing NETosis and its subsequent response are not well understood, as compared with the response after removal of either apoptotic or necrotic neutrophils by phagocytes.

Apoptotic cells impose suppressive effect on LPS-induced cytokine production of IL-1β, IL-6, and TNF-α whereas uptake of NETs promotes the LPS-induced production of these cytokines (Kobayashi, 2015). TGF-β, an antiinflammatory cytokine, is produced when apoptotic cells get ingested by macrophages but not always. Upon interaction of macrophages with apoptotic cells nitric oxide (NO) is produced which leads to down modulation of neutrophil-specific chemokine (MIP-2) production in vitro as well as in vivo (Shibata, Nagata, & Kobayashi, 2007). High levels of inflammatory cytokines in autoimmune patients stimulate neutrophils toward NETosis, whereas autoantibodies prompt the neutrophils to switch from apoptosis to NETosis.

NETs are generated by adherent neutrophils challenged with apoptotic cells. Filaments of decondensed chromatin decorated with bioactive molecules that are involved in the capture of various microbes and in persistent sterile inflammation. On the contrary, neutrophils that have earlier phagocytosed apoptotic cells, fail to upregulate β2 integrins and to react to stimuli that induce NET, such as IL-8. Dysregulation of NET formation contribute to the relentless inflammation and tissue injury in diseases like systemic lupus erythematosus (SLE) and AAV in which the clearance of apoptotic cells is vulnerable (Manfredi, Covino, Rovere-Querini, & Maugeri, 2015).

Necrosis in NETosis

In contrast to apoptosis, necrosis is often considered to be an unregulated and accidental cell death. However, the identification of programmed necrosis supported the existence of multiple nonapoptotic regulated cell death mechanisms. Several types of programmed necrosis have been reported, including necroptosis (Galluzzi et al., 2012), parthanatos (Xu et al., 2016), ferroptosis (Shimada et al., 2016), pyroptosis (Abe & Morrell, 2016), and NETosis (Dwivedi & Radic, 2014). Necroptosis is a type of regulated necrotic cell death that converges on a number of significant signaling pathways with apoptosis. On the whole, major understanding about necroptosis comes from studies on TNF signaling. TNF is a pleiotropic cytokine that plays a key role in the process of inflammation (Popa, Netea, Van Riel, van der Meer, & Stalenhoef, 2007). Under certain conditions, TNF acts as an effective cell death inducer through binding to TNFR. Even though there was a report that TNF-induced RIPK1-mediates caspase-independent cell death (Vercammen et al., 1998), TNF-induced nonapoptotic cell death did not fascinate enough, until researchers discovered that cells undergo necrosis-like death when apoptosis was blocked (Degterev et al., 2005; Degterev et al., 2008).

After leaving the peripheral circulation most neutrophils undergo apoptosis even in absence of infection. When apoptosis advances in an organized manner, apoptotic bodies which include potentially injurious granular enzymes are engulfed by tissue macrophages and other phagocytes. On the other hand, necrosis is a chaotic cell death. Toxic component like proteolytic enzymes and oxidant-generating enzymes are released from the necrotic cells in an unregulated manner when triggered by unexpected events. During infection, perhaps neutrophil necrosis is one of the reasons behind tissue damage, but very scarce information is available about the mechanism through which they undergo necrosis (Biermann et al., 2016).

Response to necrosis

Damage-associated molecular patterns (DAMPs) (Matzinger, 2002) are released by necrotic cells which includes high-mobility group box 1 (HMGB1) (Scaffidi, Misteli, & Bianchi, 2002), heat shock proteins, uric acid, DNA−chromatin complexes, and antimicrobial peptides which are recognized by specific receptors, PRRs and stimulate the synthesis of pro-inflammatory mediators. HMGB1 released from the necrotic cells stimulates inflammatory cytokine secretion by monocytes and regulates gene transcription (Scaffidi et al., 2002). DNA−chromatin complexes and heat shock proteins (HSPs) are also known to stimulate production of pro-inflammatory cytokines.

As PRRs have been known to recognize the molecular patterns of microorganisms and their associated products via pathogen-associated molecular patterns (PAMPs) like LPS, peptidoglycan, and flagellin, which are of bacterial origin, as well as RNA and DNA, which can be of viral or bacterial origin. Among PRRs, Toll-like receptor (TLR) is well studied, and more than 10 TLR subtypes have been recognized in humans. Among them, TLR-3 senses viral double-stranded RNA, and allows macrophages to recognize necrotic neutrophils debris, leading to stimulation of pro-inflammatory cytokines secretion (Zanetti, 2004).

Morphology of necrotic neutrophils

Necrotic neutrophils are specified to have a swollen cytoplasm with an undisposed nucleus. Sequence of initial morphological changes in their nuclei includes fusion of lobulated nuclei and turning to a large round structure followed by cell inflation and membrane disintegration (Iba, Hashiguchi, Nagaoka, Tabe, & Murai, 2013). As initially many of the neutrophils undergo apoptosis these are not the primary morphological changes but in the event of severe insult. In the beginning neutrophils directed toward apoptosis pathway at time take a turn toward necrosis, and this attempt is known as "secondary necrosis" (Silva, 2010). At end of necrosis, chromatin decondensation and leakage of nuclear contents into the cytoplasm occurs leaving the nuclear membrane intact. Cell necrosis ultimately causes the permeabilization of the cytoplasmic membrane and leakage of cellular contents by autolysis (Perry, Elson, Mitchell, Andrew, & Catterall, 1994).

Necrotic injury is usually accompanied with massive neutrophil infiltration. Depending on the extent of organ damage, the resulting severity may lead to acute life-threatening conditions. Neutrophil infiltration is the crucial primary process of the inflammatory response to sterile necrosis. The concurrence of necrotic cells and NETosis leads to the entrapment of the dead cells (Azzouz et al., 2018).

Due to loss of membrane integrity in both NETosis and necrosis, intracellular proteins leak outside the cells. Even after NETosis, some of the intracellular proteins like MPO, S100A8, and S100A9 remain associated with DNA (Khandpur et al., 2013), but not others like HMGB1 and HSPs (Kaczmarek, Vandenabeele, & Krysko, 2013; Khandpur et al., 2013). Hence, it can be speculated that DAMPs like HMGB1 and HSPs are released in both NETosis and necrosis to stimulate inflammatory responses. Fig. 3.3 provides a summary of how the apoptosis, autophagy, and necrosis pathways converge into NETosis.

Various stimuli for neutrophil extracellular trap induction

The discovery that citrullination of histones by PAD4 is critical event is a landmark in the process of understanding the mechanism of NET formation (Leshner et al., 2012; Li et al., 2010; Wang et al., 2009). Even though these molecules are essential in mediating NET formation, more recent results imply that their contribution to the process is likely stimulus-specific, and context-dependent (Douda, Khan, Grasemann, & Palaniyar, 2015; Martinod et al., 2013; Parker, Dragunow, Hampton, Kettle, & Winterbourn, 2012; Parker & Winterbourn, 2012). These observations are also in tandem with the consideration that the complicated process of NET formation is not mediated by a single signaling pathway but through a complex network of molecular and cellular events. An array of stimuli including whole microbes (bacteria, viruses, fungi, and parasites), soluble molecules (microbial and host), and microcrystals of different origin (Sørensen & Borregaard, 2016; Vorobjeva & Pinegin, 2014) has been identified that stimulate NET release in PMNs. Entrapping microorganisms is although a major function of NETs but may not be the only one. Taking into account a broad range of agents triggering NETs under sterile inflammatory conditions it is most likely that NETs contribute significantly in the general inflammatory cascade, irrespective of the stimulus. Various NET inducers have been described further.

Microcrystals

With size of $1-100\,\mu\text{m}$ microcrystals are insoluble crystals that are diverse in composition and structures. Microcrystals initiate an inflammatory response by irritating phagocytes including polymorphonuclear neutrophils (PMNs). The

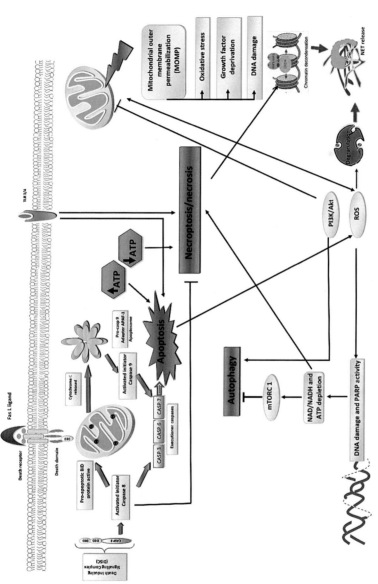

FIGURE 3.3 **Interaction of apoptosis, autophagy, and necrosis pathways during NETosis.** Binding of FasL ligand to the transmembrane death receptor recruits FADD. Receptor bound FADD forms death-inducing signaling complex (DISC) with caspase-8 which further activates executioner caspase (CASP3, CASP6, and CASP7) and proteolyze BID. BID promotes assembly of BAK-BAX leading to efflux of Cytochrome c which assembles with Apaf-1 and pro-caspase-9 forming apoptosome, which further activates the executioner caspase cascade leading to apoptosis. High level of intracellular ATP often favors apoptosis whereas low level of ATP favor necrosis. When Akt is activated, mTOR is induced to inhibit autophagy. mTOR can sense the level of intracellular ATP and relieves the inhibition of autophagy when the level of ATP is low. Activated ATP can phosphorylate certain apoptotic factors like caspase-9 leading to inhibit·on of apoptosis. Increase in ROS generation leads to DNA damage and poly (ADP-ribose) polymerase (PARP) activity causes depletion of ATP and NAD/NADH causing recrosis/necroptosis and inhibition of autophagy. ROS production also causes mitochondrial membrane permeabilization (MOMP). ROS-mediated degranulation in conjunction with necrosis-associated chromatin decondensation leads to NET release in neutrophils.

significant microcrystals involved in NET formation include gout-causing monosodium urate (MSU) crystals, pseudogout-causing calcium pyrophosphate dehydrate crystals, cholesterol crystals associated with atherosclerosis, silicosis causing silica crystals, and adjuvant alum crystals (Rada, 2017).

Monosodium urate crystals

MSU crystals are the inflammatory microcrystals that cause autoinflammatory condition, gout (Kuo, Grainge, Zhang, & Doherty, 2015). These crystals are negatively birefringent, needle shaped, and generally 5−25 μm (sometimes 100 μm) in length (Rosenthal & Mandel, 2001; Sil, Hayes, & Reaves, 2016). During nucleic acid metabolism, uric acid formed gets crystallized in the joints of gout patients. MSU crystals exaggerate the innate immune system including macrophages and PMNs, which leads to acute joint attacks that turns into chronic disease (Martinon, 2010). Activated PMN phagocytose MSU crystals and generates ROS by the NOX (Abramson, Hoffstein, & Weissmann, 1982; Gaudry et al., 1993; Naccache, Bourgoin, & Plante, 1993). The first study regarding the NET induction by MSU crystals was made by Mitroulis et al. (2011), which shows the requirement of autophagy, PI3K signaling, and endosomal acidification. As compared to healthy individuals, synovial cells and PMNs of gout patients release NETs. The gout synovial fluid and serum promote NET formation in PMNs of healthy individuals. In MSU crystal−elicited NETs histones colocalize with DNA. Basophil and eosinophil granulocytes also release NETs in response to MSU crystals along with PMNs (Schorn et al., 2012). It is proposed that similar to entrapment of bacteria, NETs also immobilize the crystals. Aggregated NETs (aggNETs) induced by MSU crystal has been shown to restrict inflammation (Schauer et al., 2014). The high concentration of PMN proteases found in aggNETs degrades several pro-inflammatory cytokines and inhibits the recruitment of new leukocytes. In vitro and in vivo formation of aggNETs vigorously reduces the amount of measurable pro-inflammatory cytokines. The deficiency of NOX2 and incompetency to form NETs causes an exacerbated, prolonged, chronic inflammation. This phenomenon can be reversed by adoptively transferring aggNETs into NETosis-deficient mice. The role of NETs has been found in gout pathogenesis (Schauer et al., 2014).

First, PMNs are recruited in large numbers to the joints of gout patients followed by encounter of MSU crystals by activated inflammasome (Maueröder, Kienhöfer, & Hahnetal, 2015). In acute gout, activation of PMNs is accompanied with inflammation-associated pain. Second, at later stages of acute attacks, at high density of PMNs, NETs form aggNETs that degrade pro-inflammatory cytokines and also densely pack crystals to stop inflammation. AggNETs were proposed to form the basis for gouty tophi (Schauer et al., 2014), a long-described white material that typically appears at the end of acute attacks and is characteristic for the chronic phase of gout

(Chhana & Dalbeth, 2015). Overall, aggNET formation was proposed to stop the acute inflammatory response at the expense of forming tophi that have been associated with symptoms of chronic gout (Maueröder et al., 2015). Regardless of the proposed novel role in gout pathogenesis, scarce information was available about the cellular and molecular mechanisms and regulation of MSU crystal−elicited NET formation but with more research input some mechanism has been figured out. PMNs of NOX2-deficient murine stimulated with MSU crystals do not release NETs and aggNETs, neither in vitro nor in vivo. Interestingly soluble uric acid stimulates NET release in a NOX-independent manner (Arai et al. 2014). Autophagy has also been proposed to mediate NET formation induced by MSU crystals and other stimuli (Mitroulis et al., 2011; Remijsen, Kuijpers et al., 2011; Remijsen, Vanden Berghe et al., 2011; Sharma, Simonson, Jondle, Mishra, & Sharma, 2017). It has been suggested by a group that NETosis is actually a PMN-specific necroptotic pathway involving RIPK1-RIPK3-MLKL signaling in MSU crystal and PMA-induced NET formation (Desai et al., 2016). This has been challenged by Amini et al. (2016) suggesting that NET release can occur independent of RIP3K and MLKL signaling, at least in response to PMA. Thus there remains a disparity in conclusion about relationship between NET formation and PMN necroptosis, hence, the need for more in-depth studies remains. PMNs do not really phagocytose MSU crystals since most of the crystals are far longer than PMNs themselves. Only a small fraction of PMNs engaged in attempting MSU crystal phagocytosis but NET releasing PMNs were all associated with MSU crystals. It can be concluded that MSU crystal phagocytosis is necessary for NET formation. It has been proposed that purinergic P2Y6 receptor is involved in this mechanism based on a strong reduction of MSU crystal−induced NET release by general purinergic receptor inhibitors and the P2Y6-specific inhibitor Mrs2578. Interestingly exonucleotides alone failed to induce NET release in human PMNs. On the other hand Mrs2578 reduced MSU crystal−stimulated ROS production, cytokine release, and PMN migration suggesting the involvement of these steps in MSU crystal promoted NET extrusion (Sil et al., 2016).

In a separate study it was revealed that IL-1β derived from macrophages enhances NET release triggered by MSU crystals (Sil, Wicklum, Surell, & Rada, 2017). IL-1β promotes NET formation but NETs degrade cytokines including IL-1β; then how these two contrasting mechanisms work in vivo in acute gout? They are most likely separated in time during the inflammatory process. While, at the early stage of gout flares, IL-1β drives inflammation, PMN recruitment and activation (pro-inflammatory segment), NETs become important later when sufficient levels accumulated and capable of aggNET formation and cytokine degradation (antiinflammatory phase). The details of this complex in vivo mechanism are, however, not well understood. Anakinra, a potent IL-1 receptor antagonist, and antibodies neutralizing IL-1β inhibit the NETosis-enhancing effect of macrophages and gout synovial fluid (Sil et al., 2017). These results add a novel mechanism by which ana-kinra works and describes IL-1β as a potentiator of NET formation linking two significant arms of the inflammatory cascade in gout, inflammasome activation in macrophages, and NET formation in PMNs, the critical role of phagocytes engulfing small urate microaggregates (SMA) in hyperuricemic blood. These SMAs form first before they grow into long, needle-shaped MSU crystals that are known to trigger NET release. Phagocytes take up SMAs and prevent the formation of MSU crystals and NETs in the circulation (Pieterse, Jeremic, & Czegley, 2016).

MSU crystals remain clinically inactive for long duration but as they get trapped in large aggNETs, inflammation ameliorates and hence, forms an amorphous material tophus, which can remain clinically inactive for long. This is the basis of granuloma formation in gout patients (Kobayashi, 2015).

Calcium pyrophosphate dihydrate crystals (CPPD)

Pseudogout also known as calcium pyrophosphate deposition disease, is a type of arthritis. It causes spontaneous, periodic acute joint attacks that potentially turn into a chronic disease with painful swelling in the joints. Pseudogout is a condition similar to gout but the causative agent is different, that is, CPPD crystals (Liu-Bryan & Liote, 2005). Compared to MSU crystals, CPPD crystals are characteristically shorter and structurally rhomboid in shape whereas MSU are needle-like crystals and they induce robust NET (Pang, Hayes, Buac, Yoo, & Rada, 2013). The morphological changes in the nuclei that occur during CPPD crystal stimulation are similar to the PMA induction. The mechanistic steps during this stimulation comprised loss of segmentation in nucleus, decondensation of nuclear material, appearance of diffuse NETs followed by full-blown NETs (Hakkim et al., 2011). For CPPD crystal−induced NET, HSP 90, PI3K, and CXCR2 activity is required whereas NOX2 activity is essential for MSU crystal−stimulated NET formation. Hence, both these crystals induce NET via different signaling pathways.

Alum

Described as the most successful adjuvant the precise mechanism of action of alum is, however, largely unknown (Exley, Siesjö, & Eriksson, 2010). The microcrystals present in the alums serve as antigen storehouse which augments the effectiveness of vaccines by increasing antigen phagocytosis on antigen presenting cells (Lambrecht, Kool, Willart, & Hammad, 2009). At the site of vaccination, PMNs are rapidly recruited which emphasize on the noteworthy alteration at the early stage of immune response. Hence, an interaction study between PMNs and adjuvants is of clinical significance (Nakayama, 2016; Oleszycka, Moran, & Tynan, 2016; Yang, Strong, Miller,

& Unanue, 2010). Upon exposure to alum crystal, PMNs release their DNA independent of ROS generation as experiments have shown that oxidase inhibitor DPI does not exhibit any effect (Warnatsch, Ioannou, Wang, & Papayannopoulos, 2015).

Cholesterol crystals

IL-1β has been found to be implicated in the pathogenesis of atherosclerosis but the mechanism by which cytokine is released by macrophage is largely unknown. For secretion of IL-1β by macrophages both PMNs and NETs are required and this will lead to recruitment of other PMNs at the site of athero-sclerotic lesions. These crystals within a concentration range stimulate NET formation in vitro in human PMNs activating inflammasome. NOX2 inhibitor DPI blocks the NET release on the other hand, cholesterol crystals stimulate the ROS generation (Warnatsch et al., 2015). During cholesterol crystal—induced NET formation neutrophil elastase (NE) is translocated in the nucleus but the PAD4 inhibitor Cl-amidine is not affected. Cholesterol crystal—induced NETs enhances cytokine release by macrophages resulting into activation of Th17 cells and augmented recruitment of leukocyte.

Silica crystals

Chronic exposure to silica crystals leads to pulmonary silicosis or chronic obstructive pulmonary disease (COPD) and is also associated with vasculitis or chronic renal failure (Hnizdoand Vallyathan, 2003; Tervaert, Stegeman, & Kallenberg, 1998). COPD is an umbrella term used to describe progressive lung diseases including emphysema, chronic bronchitis, and refractory (nonreversible) asthma. Inflammasome get activated by silica crystals and phagocytosed by immune cells including PMNs. Glomerulonephritis and small-vessel vasculitis—related NETs serve as the source of antineutrophilic cyto-plasmic antibodies (Kessenbrock et al., 2009; Yoshida, Sasaki, Sugisaki, Yamaguchi, & Yamada, 2013).

Although silica crystal stimulation of murine PMNs leads to ROS release, the in vivo relevance of this finding has not been established yet (Berlo, Wessels, & Boots, 2010). These crystal-induced NETs are concerned with lung disease (Brinkmann, Goosmann, Kühn, & Zychlinsky, 2012). In both animal models and human patients PMNs are found to be present in large numbers in the lungs in silicosis (Borges et al., 2010; Re, Dumoutier, & Couillin, 2010; Zhai et al., 2004). As compared to MSU crystals, DNA released from PMNs upon induction by silica crystals is comparable (Brinkmann et al., 2012), whereas eosinophils do not release NETs in the presence of silica crystals.

Nanoparticles

The small-sized Nanoparticles (NPs) act like adjuvants and support specific humoral and cellular immune responses by activating inflammatory reactions and tissue damage NPs are particles of size ranging between 1 and 100nm and are made up of carbon, metal, metal oxides, or organic matter (Hasan, 2015). They display unique physical, chemical, and biological properties at nanoscale in contrast to their respective particles at higher scales. This happens due to a relatively larger surface area to the volume, increased reactivity or stability in a chemical process, enhanced mechanical strength, etc. These properties of NPs have led to their use in various applications. NPs differ in their dimensions, shapes, and sizes apart from their material (Cho et al., 2013). NP can be either a zero dimensional where the length, breadth, and height is fixed at a single point, for example, nano dots; one dimension where it can possess only one parameter, for example, graphene; two dimension where it has length and breadth, for example, carbon nano-tubes or three dimension where it has all the parameters such as length, breadth, and height, for example, gold NPs. NPs are of different shape, size, and structure. It may be spherical, cylindrical, tubular, conical, hollow core, spiral, flat, or irregular. The surface can be a uniform or irregular with surface variations. Some NPs are crystalline or amorphous with single or multi crystal solids either loose or agglomerated (Machado, Pacheco, Nouws, Albergaria, & Delerue-Matos, 2015).

Earlier the research concerned with the exposure of neutrophils to nano-materials was focused on studies related to cytotoxicity, phagocytic uptake, and degranulation. After that nanodiamonds were found to induce necrosis and self-limited sterile inflammation. These nanostructures induce NETosis in cultured neutrophils (Biermann et al., 2016).

The size of NPs is crucial for determining NETosis and this is related with the resolution of an initial neutrophil-driven inflammation in air pouches. Size plays an important role as in vitro granulocytes do not take up microdiamonds of 1 µm, whereas small nanodiamonds induced NETosis due to their smaller size and hydrophobicity. These NPs vary to a great extent in size and properties as compared to pathogens like bacteria or yeast, hence, neutrophils respond differently to pathogens than nanodiamonds. As nanodia-monds cause extensive cellular damage in vitro and remain at the site of injection, it can be assumed that they provoke chronic inflammation after in vivo injection.

The size for strong interaction of hydrophobic particles with phospholipid bilayers has been expected to be 10 nm. Because of the ample presence of nonpolar NPs in the environment, it is important to study the ability of living beings to entrap NPs via formation of NETs. When NPs of size ranging in between 10 and 40 nm interact with the various cell types and tissues they induce fast (<20 min) damage of plasma membranes and lysosomal compartment loses its stability altogether leading to the immediate formation of NETs. On the other hand, particles sized between 100 and 1000 nm are inert. Persistence of small NPs in joints caused unremitting arthritis and bone remodeling. Small NPs coinjected with antigen exerted adjuvant-like activity (Muñoz et al., 2016). There is no information available regarding uptake of NPs by neutrophils through specific receptor. NPs having higher hydrophobicity directly interact with lipids of cell membranes.

While RBCs are exposed to nanodiamonds of different sizes they cause increase in granularity of the cells along with the damage to erythrocyte membranes is not attributable to activation of the complement system because all NPs activated the complement cascade to the same extent and regardless of their size (Muñoz et al., 2016).

An immediate inflammatory response commences with entrapment of NPs in NETs which is endowed with an intrinsic mechanism for the resolution of inflammation. External and internal cellular membrane barrier and the property of ion selectivity get disturbed with the induction of small-sized NPs. Therefore it leads to release of low molecular weight mediators between the cellular compartments. After damage membranes are engulfed for recycling and fuse with primary lysosomes, phagolysosome form. Increase in ROS production and further activation of intracellular pathways, finally lead to decondensation and externalization of chromatin. To deal with NPs intruding natural barriers, body adapts two strategies, one in the lungs and another in the tissues. In the lung, mononuclear phagocytes take up NPs at once and clear them within 2 weeks without inducing signs of explicit inflammation. On the contrary, NPs are immobilized in the body tissues by interstitial aggNETs. The containment of the NPs in these aggNETs and the proteolytical degradation of pro-inflammatory mediators by NET-bound serine proteases temporally and spatially restrict the initial response and orchestrate the resolution of local inflammation (Muñoz et al., 2016).

Silver nanoparticles (AgNPs) with an initial diameter of 20 nm induce apoptosis in human neutrophils (Poirier, Simard, Antoine, & Girard, 2014). AgNP of size 15 nm causes cell death in human PMNs by a mechanism that involves the inflammatory caspase-1 and -4 and also ROS generation. However, AgNP15 induced NET release is not reversed by caspase-1 and -4 inhibitors and by the antioxidant n-acetylcysteine (Simard et al., 2015).

NET formation under hypoxic condition

In the life cycle of aerobic organisms, oxygen (O_2) is an indispensable element. The central role of oxygen is due to the fact that it is the final acceptor of electrons in the mitochondrial respiratory chain. This allows the process of oxidative phosphorylation and the generation of cellular energy, in the form of ATP, to ensue. ATP is involved in carrying out most of the reactions that are necessary to maintain cellular viability (Hardie, 2003; Lopez-Barneo,

Pardal, & Ortega-Saenz, 2001). To survive under normoxia, a cell continuously maintains a high and constant ratio of cellular ATP/ADP ratio. The dependence of cells on a high constant ATP/ADP ratio means a dependence on oxygen. A reduction in the level of normal oxygen supply is called hypoxia and this will have impact on the cell viability. Hypoxia is encountered not only in different conditions including the patho-physiological conditions, such as atherosclerosis, obstructive sleep apnea, mountain sickness, ischemic diseases (stroke) and cancer, but also in physiological processes, such as embryonic development (Brahimi-Horn, Chiche, & Pouyssegur, 2007; Brahimi-Horn & Pouyssegu, 2007; Li et al., 2006; Sluimer et al., 2008). Various terms have been used in regard to the reduction of oxygen supply. The term hypoxemia is defined as a reduced oxygenation of the blood. Hypoxia is defined as a decrease in the oxygen supply to a level insufficient to maintain cellular function. Hypoxia−ischemia stands for the processes of hypoxia combined with ischemia. Ischemia differs from hypoxia as it is not only a decrease in the oxygen supply but also involves a reduction of the blood flow leading to decreased nutrient supply and accumulation of metabolic products like carbon dioxide, lactic acid and ammonia (Biagas, 1999; Sharp et al., 2004). Additionally, hypoxia response can be divided into different time scales: an acute, an intermediate, and a chronic response (Fig. 3.4), and different levels of oxygen concentration: a moderate (5%−8% O_2) and an anoxic level (<1 O_2) (normoxia is 21% O_2). The brain is regarded as the most hypoxia-sensitive organ because of its need for a high oxygen supply, whereas the skeletal muscle is among the most hypoxia-tolerant.

Cellular effects of hypoxia

There have been few studies on evaluating the effect of hypoxia on NET formation and there are variations in the findings. Some studies have shown that hypoxia increases NETs formation (Fig. 3.4) and adhesion to endothelial cells. Expression of adhesion molecule in human umbilical vein endothelial cells (HUVECs), neutrophil adherence to HUVEC monolayers, and NETosis are modulated by switching to hypoxia (Khawaja et al., 2015). NET formation has also been seen to increase in intratumoral hypoxia in metastatic tumors (Tohme et al., 2016). However, in an another study by Branitzki-Heinemann et al. (2016), it was found that PMA-induced neutrophils show significantly reduced NET formation. However, S. aureas−induced NET formation was unaffected compared to normoxia conditions suggesting that different stimulus may have a different impact of NET induction during hypoxia.

Hypoxia increases NETosis

During infection or inflammation, there is overconsumption of oxygen by pathogens and immune cells recruitment which causes hypoxia.

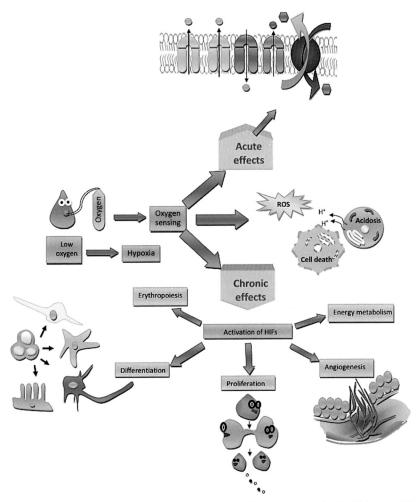

FIGURE 3.4 Cellular effects of hypoxia. Oxygen supply decreases to a level which is insufficient to maintain cellular function. This leads to certain critical responses that can either be acute or chronic. Acute response can disturb the ionic homeostasis. The chronic response involves activation and stabilization of hypoxia-inducible factors (HIFs). HIFs regulate the genes involved in erythropoietin. The expression of erythropoietin gene increases during hypoxia, enhancing the delivery of oxygen to tissue. HIF-1 also activates VEGF, TGF-β, and angiopoietin which are involved in angiogenesis. ATP generation by oxidative phosphorylation is arrested during hypoxia. HIF also regulates the glucose metabolism. Cell differentiation in number of cells is enhanced during hypoxia. HIFs have association with the molecules that are critical for the regulation of differentiation of the cells, including notch, oct-4, and MYC. Sudden growth factors like TGF-α and IGF-2 are HIF-1 target genes which activate signal transduction pathways leading to the cell proliferation and survival. Cellular pH homostasis gets disturbed during hypoxia leading to acidosis. HIF-1 induces the Bcl-2 family leading to cell death. Hence these all show various cellular responses during hypoxia in order to combat and to maintain the oxygen homeostasis.

Hypoxia-inducible factor 1α (HIF-1α) regulates the induced hypoxia condition. HIF-1α is stabilized by the iron chelating HIF-1α-agonist desferoxamine or AKB-4924 enhancing the release of phagocyte extracellular traps (Fig. 3.5).

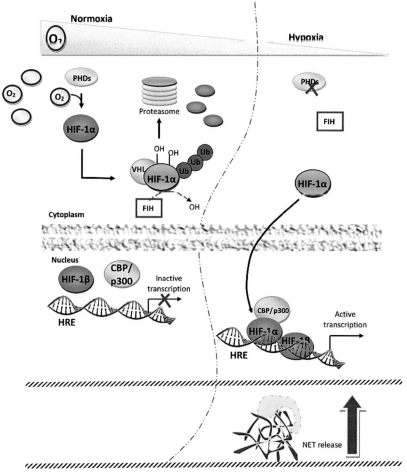

FIGURE 3.5   Hypoxia increases NETosis. During normoxia, HIF-1α is hydroxylated by oxygen sensitive prolyl hydroxylase domain (PHD) proteins which then interact with the ubiquitin E3-containing ligase von hippellindau complex (pVHL). By this HIF-1α is targeted for proteasomal degradation. HIF-1α is hydroxylated by factor inhibiting HIF-1α (FIH-1) which is oxygen sensitive enzyme, inhibits interaction with the transcriptional coactivator CBP/p300 repressing transactivation activity of HIF-1. Whereas, during hypoxia the PHDs and the FIH-1 become inactive which leads to dimerization of HIF-1α with HIF-1β, this heterodimer translocates to nucleus and binds to HRE present on target genes. CBP/p300 is recruited as FIH-1 is inactive and activated the transcription. Increase in NETosis has been observed during hypoxia.

There are major changes in the level of oxygen in between arterial and venous circulations which are faced by neutrophils. The cells that are located far from capillaries survive in a condition of "physiological hypoxia." Infection and inflammation exhibit a condition of "pathological hypoxia." While neutrophil chemotaxis and phagocytosis are preserved under conditions of profound hypoxia, the ability to mount an oxidative burst and consequent killing of organisms, such as *S. aureus*, are markedly impaired (McGovern et al., 2011). Since neutrophil-derived proteases play such a key role in the pathogenesis of COPD (Hoenderdos & Condliffe, 2013) and cystic fibrosis (Garratt, Sutanto, & Ling, 2015), and local tissue hypoxia is highly relevant to airway inflammation in these conditions.

Activated HIF-1α-mediated NF-$\kappa\beta$ inhibits apoptosis which results into enhanced neutrophil survival. The release of all major neutrophil granule population is upregulated under hypoxia condition which leads to damage of respiratory epithelial cells in vitro. This is not mediated by HIF-1α, but is due to enhanced basal and cytokine-stimulated neutrophil AKT phosphorylation. PI3Kγ plays an important role in hypoxia-enhanced degranulation. Neutrophils behave differently under the conditions of hypoxia and normoxia which emphasize the significance of physiological oxygen level in context to neutrophil functions (Lanzen et al., 2006).

Role of pH in neutrophil extracellular trap induction

The acidification of local surrounding is a general feature in human pathologies, such as tumor and inflammation. The resulting change in pH conditions alters the, immune cell's functions. The extracellular acidification turns out to be a vital modulator of innate immunity. Under the acidic environment, neutrophil apoptosis is delayed, respiratory burst is inhibited, amplified polarization, altered chemotaxis, enhanced endocytosis, and suppressed killing bacteria. It has been found that the immune response of neutrophils can be altered by the change of extracellular pH (Kellum, Song, & Li, 2004; Lardner, 2001). The acidification of local environment is a common feature under some pathological conditions. The extracellular acidification is associated with the process of inflammation, and the pH value of the microenvironment becomes 5.5–7.0 (Van Hoogmoed et al., 1999; Latson, Nieto, Beldomenico, & Snyder, 2005; Simmen & Blaser, 1993). Such changes in the extracellular pH may bring noteworthy alterations in the immune response. Studies show that extracellular acidification may alter the release of inflammatory mediator, and various kinds of acids at specific pH value can cause a different change. Besides that, extracellular acidification also plays a significant role in modulating the function of immune cells, including polymorphonuclear leukocytes, macrophages, and lymphocytes (López et al., 1999). Upon migration from the blood to the nearby tissues, neutrophils encounter changes in extracellular pH (pH$_e$) conditions. Activated NOX2 causes increased concentration of H^+ ions leading to reduced intracellular pH (pH_i). It is proposed that NETosis is stimulated with increase in pH which leads to increase in NOX-mediated ROS generation along with neutrophil protease activity. With increase in pH_e, pH_i of both activated and resting neutrophils increases. As compared to resting neutrophils, activated ones are having lower pH_i because there is increased concentration of H^+ ions due to NOX activity. Induction of NETosis with PMA results in increased NOX-dependent ROS generation due to higher pH. Increased pH stimulates histone H4 cleavage as well as NETosis in activated neutrophils. Higher pH_e supports NOX-dependent ROS production, protease activity, and NETosis and vice-versa. Raising pH either by sodium bicarbonate or Tris base (clinically known as Tris hydroxymethyl aminomethane, tromethamine, or THAM) increases NETosis, hence pH regulates NET formation. The amount of Tris solution required to increase the pH is less than that of equimolar bicarbonate solution as one molecule of Tris can bind to $3H^+$ ions, contrary to this, each bicarbonate (HCO_3^-) ion binds $1H^+$ ion (Khan et al., 2018).

It is not yet well understood how pH impacts calcium-dependent NOX-independent NET formation. The mechanistic steps of NOX-independent NET formation involve calcium influx, mitochondrial reactive oxygen species (mROS) generation, and histone citrullination along with histone cleavage. Rise in pH influences calcium-dependent NOX-independent NETosis. A slight increase in pH significantly increases intracellular calcium concentration in resting and stimulated neutrophils, respectively. Like calcium, mROS generation also increases with increase in pH. Little or no histone cleavage was noted in unstimulated cells, at any pH. Both histone citrullination (CitH3) and cleavage of histones facilitate DNA decondensation. Therefore, increase in pH increases PAD4 activity as can be assessed by the CitH3 and histone cleavage (de Souza et al., 2018). In contrast to calcium ionophores, pH-dependent histone cleavage is higher when NETosis is inducted by ionomycin. At any pH, unstimulated cells show very low or not any histone cleavage.

References

Abe, J., & Morrell, C. (2016). Pyroptosis as a regulated form of necrosis: PI^+/annexin V^-/high caspase 1/low caspase 9 activity in cells = pyroptosis? *Circulation Research, 118*, 1457−1460.

Abramson, S., Hoffstein, S. T., & Weissmann, G. (1982). Superoxide anion generation by human neutrophils exposed to monosodium urate. Effect of protein adsorption and complement activation. *Arthritis and Rheumatology, 25*, 174−180.

Amini, P., Stojkov, D., Wang, X., Wicki, S., Kaufmann, T., Wong, W. W., ... Yousefi, S. (2016). NET formation can occur independently of RIPK3 and MLKL signalling. *European Journal of Immunology, 46*, 178−184.

Arai, Y., Nishinaka, Y., Arai, T., Morita, M., Mizugishi, K., Adachi, S., ... Yamashita, K. (2014). Uric acid induces NADPH oxidase-independent neutrophil extracellular trap formation. *Biochemical and Biophysical Research Communications, 443*, 556−561.

Arcaro, A., & Wymann, M. P. (1993). Wortmannin is a potent phosphatidylinositol 3-kinase inhibitor: The role of phosphatidylinositol 3,4,5-trisphosphate in neutrophil responses. *Biochemical Journal, 296*, 297−301.

Azzouz, D., Khan, M. A., Sweezey, N., & Palaniyar, N. (2018). Two-in-one: UV radiation simultaneously induces apoptosis and NETosis. *Cell Death Discovery, 4*, 51.

Babior, B. M. (1999). NADPH oxidase: An update. *Blood, 93*, 1464−1476.

Berlo, D. V., Wessels, A., & Boots, A. W. (2010). Neutrophil-derived ROS contribute to oxidative DNA damage induction by quartz particles. *Free Radical Biology and Medicine, 49*, 1685−1693.

Biagas, K. (1999). Hypoxic-ischemic brain injury: Advancements in the understanding of mechanisms and potential avenues for therapy. *Current Opinion in Pediatrics, 11*, 223−228.

Bianchi, M., Hakkim, A., Brinkmann, V., Siler, U., Seger, R. A., Zychlinsky, A., & Reichenbach, J. (2009). Restoration of NET formation by gene therapy in CGD controls aspergillosis. *Blood, 114*, 2619−2622.

Biermann, M. H. C., Podolska, M. J., Knopf, J., Reinwald, C., Weidner, D., Maueröder, C., & Munoz, L. E. (2016). Oxidative burst-dependent NETosis is implicated in the resolution of necrosis-associated sterile inflammation. *Frontiers in Immunology, 7*, 1−13.

Blommaart, E. F., Krause, U., Schellens, J. P., Vreeling-Sindelárová, H., & Meijer, A. J. (1997). The phosphatidylinositol 3-kinase inhibitors wortmannin and LY294002 inhibit autophagy in isolated rat hepatocytes. *European Journal of Biochemistry, 15*, 240−246.

Brahimi-Horn, M. C., Chiche, J., & Pouyssegur, J. (2007). Hypoxia signaling control metabolic demand. *Current Opinion in Cell Biology, 19*, 223−229.

Brahimi-Horn, M. C., & Pouyssegu, J. (2007). Oxygen, a source of life and stress. *FEBS Letters, 581*, 3582−3591.

Branitzki-Heinemann, K., Möllerherm, H., Völlger, L., Husein, D. M., de Buhr, N., Blodkamp, S., & von Köckritz-Blickwede, M. (2016). Formation of neutrophil extracellular traps under low oxygen level. *Frontiers in Immunology., 7*, 518.

Brinkmann, V., Goosmann, C., Kühn, L. I., & Zychlinsky, A. (2012). Automatic quantification of in vitro NET formation. *Frontiers in Immunology, 3*, 413.

Brinkmann, V., Reichard, U., Goosmann, C., Fauler, B., Uhlemann, Y., Weiss, D. S., ... Zychlinsky, A. (2004). Neutrophil extracellular traps kill bacteria. *Science, 303*, 1532−1535.

Brinkmann, V., & Zychlinsky, A. (2007). Beneficial suicide: Why neutrophils die to make NETs. *Nature Reviews Microbiology, 5*, 577−582.

Chen, Q., Kang, J., & Fu, C. (2018). The independence of and associations among apoptosis, autophagy, and necrosis. *Signal Transduction and Targeted Therapy, 3*(1), 18. Available from https://doi.org/10.1038/s41392-018-0018-5.

Chhana, A., & Dalbeth, N. (2015). The gouty tophus: A review. *Current Rheumatology Reports, 17*, 3.

Clemmensen, S. N., Bohr, C. T., Rørvig, S., Glenthøj, A., Mora-Jensen, H., & Cramer, E. P. (2012). Olfactomedin 4 defines a subset of human neutrophils. *Journal of Leukocyte Biology, 91*, 495−500.

Croker, B. A., O Donnell, J. A., Nowell, C. J., Metcalf, D., Dewson, G., Campbell, K. J., ... Roberts, A. W. (2011). Fas-mediated neutrophil apoptosis is accelerated by Bid, Bak, and Bax and inhibited by Bcl-2 and Mcl-1. *Proceedings of the National Academy of Sciences of the United States of America, 108*, 13135−13140.

deCathelineau, A. M., & Henson, P. M. (2003). The final step in programmed cell death: Phagocytes carry apoptotic cells to the grave. *Essays in Biochemistry, 39*, 105.

Degterev, A., Hitomi, J., Germscheid, M., Ch'en, I. L., Korkina, O., Teng, X., ... Yuan, J. (2008). Identification of RIP1 kinase as a specific cellular target of necrostatins. *Nature Chemical Biology, 4*, 313–321.

Degterev, A., Huang, Z., Boyce, M., Li, Y., Jagtap, P., Mizushima, N., ... Yuan, J. (2005). Chemical inhibitor of nonapoptotic cell death with therapeutic potential for ischemic brain injury. *Nature Chemical Biology, 1*, 112–119.

de Souza, C. N., Breda, L. C. D., Khan, M. A., de Almeida, S. R., Câmara, N. O. S., Sweezey, N., & Palaniyar, N. (2018). Alkaline pH promotes NADPH oxidase-independent neutrophil extracellular trap formation: A matter of mitochondrial reactive oxygen species generation and citrullination and cleavage of histone. *Frontiers in Immunology,, 8,* 1–15

Desai, J., Kumar, S. V., Mulay, S. R., Konrad, L., Romoli, S., Schauer, C., ... Anders, H. J. (2016). PMA and crystal- induced neutrophil extracellular trap formation involves RIPK1-RIPK3-MLKL signalling. *European Journal of Immunology, 46*, 223–229.

DeSouza-Vieira, T., Costa, A. G., Rochael, N. C., Lira, M. N., Nascimento, M. T., Lima-Gomez, P. S., ... Saraiva, E. M. (2016). Neutrophil extracellular traps release induced by Leishmania: Role of PI3Kgamma, ERK, PI3Ksigma, PKC, and [Ca^{2+}]. *Journal of Leukocyte Biology, 100*, 801–810.

Douda, D. N., Khan, M. A., Grasemann, H., & Palaniyar, N. (2015). SK3 channel and mitochondrial ROS mediate NADPH oxidase-independent NETosis induced by calcium influx. *Proceedings of the National Academy of Sciences of the United States of America, 112*, 2817–2822.

Dwivedi, N., & Radic, M. (2014). Citrullination of autoantigens implicates NETosis in the induction of autoimmunity. *Annals of the Rheumatic Diseases, 73*, 483–491.

Exley, C., Siesjö, P., & Eriksson, H. (2010). The immunobiology of aluminium adjuvants: How do they really work? *Trends in Immunology, 31*, 103–109.

Fuchs, T. A., Abed, U., Goosmann, C., Hurwitz, R., Schulze, I., & Wahn, V. (2007). Novel cell death program leads to neutrophil extracellular traps. *Journal of Cell Biology, 176*, 231–241.

Galluzzi, L., Vitale, I., Abrams, J. M., Alnemri, E. S., Baehrecke, E. H., Blagosklonny, M. V., ... Kroemer, G. (2012). Molecular definitions of cell death subroutines: Recommendations of the Nomenclature Committee on Cell Death 2012. *Cell death and Differentiation, 19*, 107–120.

Garratt, L. W., Sutanto, E. N., & Ling, K. M. (2015). Matrix metalloproteinase activation by free neutrophil elastase contributes to bronchiectasis progression in early cystic fibrosis. *European Respiratory Journal, 46*, 384–394.

Gaudry, M., Roberge, C. J., De Medicis, R., Lussier, A., Poubelle, P. E., & Naccache, P. H. (1993). Crystal-induced neutrophil activation. III. Inflammatory microcrystals induce a distinct pattern of tyrosine phosphorylation in human neutrophils. *Journal of Clinical Investigation, 91*, 1649–1655.

Hakkim, A., Fuchs, T. A., Martinez, N. E., Hess, S., Prinz, H., Zychlinsky, A., & Waldmann, H. (2011). Activation of the Raf-MEK-ERK pathway is required for neutrophil extracellular trap formation. *Nature Chemical Biology, 7*, 75–77.

Hardie, D. G. (2003). Minireview: The AMP-activated protein kinase cascade: The key sensor of cellular energy status. *Endocrinology., 144*, 5179–5183.

Hasan, S. (2015). A review on nanoparticles: Their synthesis and types. *Research Journal of Recent Sciences, 4*, 9–11.

Hnizdo, E., & Vallyathan, V. (2003). Chronic obstructive pulmonary disease due to occupational exposure to silica dust: A review of epidemiological and pathological evidence. *Occupational and Environmental Medicine, 60*, 237–243.

Hoenderdos, K., & Condliffe, A. (2013). The neutrophil in chronic obstructive pulmonary disease. *The American Journal of Respiratory Cell and Molecular Biology, 48,* 531−539.

Iba, T., Hashiguchi, N., Nagaoka, I., Tabe, Y., & Murai, M. (2013). Neutrophil cell death in response to infection and its relation to coagulation. *Journal of Intensive Care, 1,* 1−10.

Itakura, A., & McCarty, O. J. (2013). Pivotal role for the mTOR pathway in the formation of neutrophil extracellular traps via regulation of autophagy. *American Journal of Physiology-Cell Physiology, 305,* C348−C354.

Jia, S. H., Parodo, J., Kapus, A., Rotstein, O. D., & Marshall, J. C. (2008). Dynamic regulation of neutrophil survival through tyrosine phosphorylation or dephosphorylation of caspase-8. *Journal of Biological Chemistry, 283,* 5402−5413.

Kaczmarek, A., Vandenabeele, P., & Krysko, D. (2013). Necroptosis: The release of damage-associated molecular patterns and its physiological relevance. *Immunity., 38,* 209−223.

Kellum, J. A., Song, M., & Li, J. (2004). Science review: Extracellular acidosis and the immune response: Clinical and physiologic implications. *Critical Care., 8,* 331−336.

Kessenbrock, K., Krumbholz, M., & Schönermarck, U. (2009). Netting neutrophils in autoimmune small-vessel vasculitis. *Nature Medicine, 15,* 623−625.

Khan, M. A., Philip, L. M., Cheung, G., Vadakepeedika, S., Grasemann, H., Sweezey, N., & Palaniyar, N. (2018). Regulating NETosis: increasing pH promotes NADPH oxidase-dependent NETosis. *Frontiers of Medicine., 5,* 1−19.

Khandpur, R., Carmona-Rivera, C., Vivekanandan-Giri, A., Gizinski, A., Yalavarthi, S., Knight, J. S., ... Kaplan, M. J. (2013). NETs are a source of citrullinated autoantigens and stimulate inflammatory responses in rheumatoid arthritis. *Science Translational Medicine, 5,* 178ra40.

Khawaja, A. A., Pericleous, C., Thomas, L. W., Ashcroft, M., Porter, J. C., & Giles, I. (2015). Hypoxia increases neutrophil extracellular trap formation and adhesion to endothelial cells. *Rheumatology, 54,* i41−i42.

Klionsky, D. J., & Emr, S. D. (2000). Autophagy as a regulated pathway of cellular degradation. *Science., 290,* 1717−1721.

Kobayashi, Y. (2015). Neutrophil biology: An update. *EXCLI Journal., 14,* 220−227.

Kuo, C. F., Grainge, M. J., Zhang, W., & Doherty, M. (2015). Global epidemiology of gout: Prevalence, incidence and risk factors. *Nature Reviews Rheumatology, 11,* 649−662.

Lambrecht, B. N., Kool, M., Willart, M. A., & Hammad, H. (2009). Mechanism of action of clinically approved adjuvants. *Current Opinion in Immunology, 21,* 23−29.

Lanzen, J., Braun, R. D., Klitzman, B., Brizel, D., Secomb, T. W., & Dewhirst, M. W. (2006). Direct demonstration of instabilities in oxygen concentrations within the extravascular compartment of an experimental tumour. *Cancer Research., 66,* 2219−2223.

Lardner, A. (2001). The effects of extracellular pH on immune function. *Journal of Leukocyte Biology, 4,* 522−530.

Latson, K. M., Nieto, J. E., Beldomenico, P. M., & Snyder, J. R. (2005). Evaluation of peritoneal fluid lactate as a marker of intestinal ischaemia in equine colic. *Equine Veterinary Journal, 37,* 342−346.

Leshner, M., Wang, S., Lewis, C., Zheng, H., Chen, X. A., Santy, L., & Wang, Y. (2012). PAD4 mediated histone hypercitrullination induces heterochromatin decondensation and chromatin unfolding to form neutrophil extracellular trap-like structures. *Frontiers in Immunology, 3,* 307.

Li, J., Bosch-Marce, M., Nanayakkara, A., Savransky, V., Fried, S. K., Semenza, G. L., & Polotsky, V. Y. (2006). Altered metabolic responses to intermittent hypoxia in mice with partial deficiency of hypoxia-inducible factor-1α. *Physiological Genomics., 25,* 450−457.

Li, P., Li, M., Lindberg, R. M., Kennett, M. J., Xiong, N., & Wang, Y. (2010). PAD4 is essential for antibacterial innate immunity mediated by neutrophil extracellular traps. *Journal of Experimental Medicine, 207*, 1853−1862.

Liu, M., Wilk, S. A., Wang, A., Zhou, L., Wang, R. H., Ogawa, W., ... Liu, F. (2010). Resveratrol inhibits mTOR signaling by promoting the interaction between mTOR and DEPTOR. *Journal of Biological Chemistry., 285*(47), 36387−36394. Available from https://doi.org/10.1074/jbc.M110.169284, Epub 2010 Sep 17. PubMed PMID: 20851890; PubMed Central PMCID: PMC2978567.

Liu-Bryan, R., & Liote, F. (2005). Monosodium urate and calcium pyrophosphate dihydrate (CPPD) crystals, inflammation, and cellular signalling. *Joint Bone Spine, 72*, 295   302.

López, D. H., Trevani, A. S., Salamone, G., Andonegui, G., Raiden, S., & Giordano, M. (1999). Acidic pH increases the avidity of FcγR for immune complexes. *Immunology, 98*, 450−455.

Lopez-Barneo, J., Pardal, R., & Ortega-Saenz, P. (2001). Cellular mechanism of oxygen sensing. *Annual Review of Physiology, 63*, 259−287.

Ma, R., Li, T., Cao, M., Si, Y., Wu, X., Zhao, L., ... Shi, J. (2016). Extracellular DNA traps released by acute promyelocytic leukemia cells through autophagy. *Cell Death & Disease, 7*, 186.

Machado, S., Pacheco, J. G., Nouws, H. P. A., Albergaria, J. T., & Delerue-Matos, C. (2015). Characterization of green zero-valent iron nanoparticles produced with tree leaf extracts. *Science of the Total Environment, 533*, 76−81.

Mantredi, A. A., Covino, C., Rovere-Querini, P., & Maugeri, N. (2015). Instructive influences of phagocytic clearance of dying cells on neutrophil extracellular trap generation. *Clinical and Experimental Immunology, 179*, 24−29.

Martinod, K., Demers, M., Fuchs, T. A., Wong, S. L., Brill, A., Gallant, M., ... Wagner, D. D. (2013). Neutrophil histone modification by peptidyl arginine deiminase 4 is critical for deep vein thrombosis in mice. *Proceedings of the National Academy of Sciences of the United States of America, 110*, 8674−8679.

Martinon, F. (2010). Update on biology: Uric acid and the activation of immune and inflammatory cell. *Current Rheumatology Reports, 12*, 135−141.

Matzinger, P. (2002). The danger model: A renewed sense of self. *Science., 296*, 301−305.

Maueröder, C., Kienhöfer, D., & Hahnetal, J. (2015). How neutrophil extracellular traps orchestrate the local immune response in gout. *Journal of Molecular Medicine, 93*, 727−734.

McGovern, N. N., Cowburn, A. S., Porter, L., Walmsley, S. R., Summers, C., Thompson, A. A. R., ... Chilvers, E. R. (2011). Hypoxia selectively inhibits respiratory burst activity and killing of Staphylococcus aureus in human neutrophils. *Journal of Immunology., 186*, 453−463.

McInturff, A. M., Cody, M. J., Elliott, E. A., Glenn, J. W., Rowley, J. W., Rondina, M. T., & Yost, C. C. (2012). Mammalian target of rapamycin regulates neutrophil extracellular trap formation via induction of hypoxia-inducible factor 1 alpha. *Blood., 120*, 3118−3125.

Medina, C. B., & Ravichandran, K. S. (2016). Do not let death do us part: "find-me" signals in communication between dying cells and the phagocytes. *Cell Death and Differentiation, 23*, 979−989.

Mitroulis, I., Kambas, K., Chrysanthopoulou, A., Skendros, P., Apostolidou, E., Kourtzelis, I., ... Ritis, K. (2011). Neutrophil extracellular trap formation is associated with IL-1beta and autophagy-related signaling in gout. *PLoS One, 6*, e29318.

Muñoz, L. E., Bilyy, R., Biermann, M. H. C., Kienhöfer, D., Maueröder, C., Hahn, J., & Herrmann, M. (2016). Nanoparticles size-dependently initiate self-limiting NETosis-driven inflammation. *Proceedings of the National Academy of Sciences of the United States of America*, *113*, E5856−E5865.

Naccache, P. H., Bourgoin, S., & Plante, E. (1993). Crystal-induced neutrophil activation. II. Evidence for the activation of a phosphatidylcholine-specific phospholipase D. *Arthritis & Rheumatology*, *36*, 117−125.

Nadesalingam, A., Chen, J. H. K., Farahvash, A., & Khan, M. A. (2018). Hypertonic saline suppresses NADPH oxidase-dependent neutrophil extracellular trap formation and promotes apoptosis. *Frontiers in Immunology*, *9*, 1−18.

Nagata, S. (2018). Apoptosis and clearance of apoptotic cells. *Annual Review of Immunology*, *36* (1), 489−517.

Nakayama, T. (2016). An inflammatory response is essential for the development of adaptive immunity-immunogenicity and immunotoxicity. *Vaccine.*, *34*, 5815−5818.

Oleszycka, E., Moran, H. B. T., & Tynan, G. A. (2016). IL-1α and inflammasome-independent IL-1β promote neutrophil infiltration following alum vaccination. *FEBS Journal*, *283*, 9−24.

Pang, L., Hayes, C. P., Buac, K., Yoo, D. G., & Rada, B. (2013). Pseudogout-associated inflammatory calcium pyrophosphate dihydrate microcrystals induce formation of neutrophil extracellular traps. *Journal of Immunology.*, *190*, 6488−6500.

Parker, H., Dragunow, M., Hampton, M. B., Kettle, A. J., & Winterbourn, C. C. (2012). Requirements for NADPH oxidase and myeloperoxidase in neutrophil extracellular trap formation differ depending on the stimulus. *Journal of Leukocyte Biology*, *92*, 841−849.

Parker, H., & Winterbourn, C. C. (2012). Reactive oxidants and myeloperoxidase and their involvement in neutrophil extracellular traps. *Frontiers in Immunology*, *3*, 424.

Perry, F. E., Elson, C. J., Mitchell, T. J., Andrew, P. W., & Catterall, J. R. (1994). Characterisation of an oxidative response inhibitor produced by *Streptococcus pneumoniae*. *Thorax.*, *49*, 676−683.

Pieterse, E., Jeremic, I., & Czegley, C. (2016). Blood-borne phagocytes internalize urate microaggregates and prevent intravascular NETosis by urate crystals. *Scientific Reports.*, *6*, 38229.

Poirier, M., Simard, J. C., Antoine, F., & Girard, D. (2014). Interaction between silver nanoparticles of 20 nm (AgNP20) and human neutrophils: Induction of apoptosis and inhibition of de novo protein synthesis by AgNP20 aggregates. *Journal of Applied Toxicology*, *34*, 404−412.

Popa, C., Netea, M. G., Van Riel, P. L., van der Meer, J. W., & Stalenhoef, A. F. (2007). The role of TNF-α in chronic inflammatory conditions, intermediary metabolism, and cardiovascular risk. *Journal of Lipid Research*, *48*, 751−762.

Rada, B. (2017). Neutrophil extracellular traps and microcrystals. *Journal of Immunology Research*, 7.

Re, S. L., Dumoutier, L., Couillin, I., et al. (2010). IL-17A-producing γδ T and Th17 lymphocytes mediate lung inflammation but not fibrosis in experimental silicosis. *Journal of Immunology.*, *184*, 6367−6377.

Remijsen, Q., Kuijpers, T. W., Wirawan, E., Lippens, S., Vandenabeele, P., & Vanden Berghe, T. (2011). Dying for a cause: NETosis, mechanisms behind an antimicrobial cell death modality. *Cell Death and Differentiation*, *18*, 581−588.

Remijsen, Q., Vanden Berghe, T., Parthoens, E., Asselbergh, B., Vandenabeele, P., & Willems, J. (2009). Inhibition of spontaneous neutrophil apoptosis by parabutoporin acts independently of NADPH oxidase inhibition but by lipid raft-dependent stimulation of Akt. *Journal of Leukocyte Biology*, *85*, 497−507.

Remijsen, Q., Vanden Berghe, T., Wirawan, E., Asselbergh, B., Parthoens, E., & De Rycke, R. (2011). Neutrophil extracellular trap cell death requires both autophagy and superoxide generation. *Cell Research.*, *21*, 290−304.

Rosenthal, A. K., & Mandel, N. (2001). Identification of crystals in synovial fluids and joint tissues. *Current Rheumatology Reports*, *3*, 11−16.

Scaffidi, P., Misteli, T., & Bianchi, M. E. (2002). Release of chromatin protein HMGB1 by necrotic cells triggers inflammation. *Nature*, *418*, 191−195.

Schauer, C., Janko, C., Munoz, L. E., Zhao, Y., Kienhöfer, D., Frey, B., . . . Herrmann, M. (2014). Aggregated neutrophil extracellular traps limit inflammation by degrading cytokines and chemokines. *Nature Medicine*, *20*, 511−517.

Schorn, C., Janko, C., Krenn, V., Zhao, Y., Munoz, L. E., Schett, G., & Herrmann, M. (2012). Bonding the foe—NETting neutrophils immobilize the pro-inflammatory monosodium urate crystals. *Frontiers in Immunology*, *3*.

Sha, L. L., Wang, H., Wang, C., Peng, H. Y., Chen, M., & Zhao, M. H. (2016). Autophagy is induced by anti-neutrophil cytoplasmic Abs and promotes neutrophil extracellular traps formation. *Innate Immunity.*, *22*(8), 658−665. Available from https://doi.org/10.1177/1753425916668981.

Sharma, A., Simonson, T. J., Jondle, C. N., Mishra, B. B., & Sharma, J. (2017). Mincle regulates autophagy to control neutrophil extracellular trap formation. *Journal of Infectious Diseases*, *215*, 1040−1048.

Sharp, F. R., Ran, R., Lu, A., Tang, Y., Strauss, K. I., Glass, T., . . . Bernaudin, M. (2004). Hypoxic preconditioning protects against ischemic brain injury. *Neuro Rx*, *1*, 26−35.

Sheppard, F. R., Kelher, M. R., Moore, E. E., McLaughlin, N. J., Banerjee, A., & Silliman, C. C. (2005). Structural organization of the neutrophil NADPH oxidase: Phosphorylation and translocation during priming and activation. *Journal of Leukocyte Biology*, *78*, 1025−1042.

Shibata, T., Nagata, K., & Kobayashi, Y. (2007). Cutting edge: A critical role of nitrogen oxide in preventing inflammation upon apoptotic cell clearance. *Journal of Immunology.*, *179*, 3407−3411.

Shimada, K., Skouta, R., Kaplan, A., Yang, W. S., Hayano, M., Dixon, S. J., . . . Stockwell, B. R. (2016). Global survey of cell death mechanisms reveals metabolic regulation of ferroptosis. *Nature Chemical Biology*, *12*, 497−503.

Sil, P., Hayes, C. P., & Reaves, B. J. (2016). P2Y6 receptor antagonist MRS2578 inhibits neutrophil activation and aggregated neutrophil extracellular trap formation induced by gout-associated monosodium urate crystals. *Journal of Immunology.*, *198*, 428−442.

Sil, P., Wicklum, H., Surell, C., & Rada, B. (2017). Macrophage- derived IL-1β enhances monosodium urate crystal-triggered NET formation. *Inflammation Research.*, *66*, 227−237.

Silva, M. T. (2010). Bacteria-induced phagocyte secondary necrosis as a pathogenicity mechanism. *Journal of Leukocyte Biology*, *88*, 885−896.

Simmen, H.-P., & Blaser, J. (1993). Analysis of pH and pO2 in abscesses, peritoneal fluid, and drainage fluid in the presence or absence of bacterial infection during and after abdominal surgery. *American Journal of Surgery*, *166*, 24−27.

Simon, H. U. (2003). Neutrophil apoptosis pathways and their modifications in inflammation. *Immunological Reviews.*, *193*, 101−110.

Simon, H. U., Yehia, A. H., & Schaffer, F. L. (2000). Role of reactive oxygen species (ROS) in apoptosis induction. *Apoptosis.*, *5*, 415−418.

Sluimer, J. C., Gasc, J. M., Wanroij, J. L. V., Kisters, N., Groeneweg, M., Sollewijn, G., . . . Bijnens, A. P. (2008). Hypoxia. Hypoxia-inducible transcription factor, and macrophages in human atherosclerotic plaques are correlated with intraplaque angiogenesis. *Journal of the American College of Cardiology*, *51*, 1258−1265.

Surh, C. D., & Sprent, J. (1994). T-cell apoptosis detected in situ during positive and negative selection in the thymus. *Nature.*, *372*, 100.

Sørensen, O. E., & Borregaard, N. (2016). Neutrophil extracellular traps—the dark side of neutrophils. *Journal of Clinical Investigation*, *126*, 1612−1620.

Tang, S., Zhang, Y., Yin, S. W., Gao, X. J., Shi, W. W., Wang, Y., . . . Zhang, J. B. (2015). Neutrophil extracellular trap formation is associated with autophagy-related signalling in ANCA-associated vasculitis. *Clinical and Experimental Immunology*, *180*, 408−418.

Tervaert, J. W. C., Stegeman, C. A., & Kallenberg, C. G. M. (1998). Silicon exposure and vasculitis. *Curr Opin Rheumatol*, *10*, 12−17.

Tohme, S. Y., Hamza, O., Al-Khafaji., Ahmed, B., Chidi, A. P., Loughran, P., . . . Tsung, A. (2016). Neutrophil Extracellular Traps Promote the Development and Progression of Liver Metastases after Surgical Stress. *Cancer Research*, *76*(6), 1367. Available from https://doi.org/10.1158/0008-5472.CAN-15-1591.

Van Hoogmoed, L., Rodger, L. D., Spier, S. J., Gardner, I. A., Yarbrough, T. B., & Snyder, J. R. (1999). Evaluation of peritoneal fluid pH, glucose concentration, and lactate dehydrogenase activity for detection of septic peritonitis in horses. *Journal of the American Veterinary Medical Association*, *214*, 1032−1036.

Vercammen, D., Beyaert, R., Denecker, G., Goossens, V., Van Loo, G., Declercq, W., . . . Vandenabeele, P. (1998). Inhibition of caspases increases the sensitivity of L929 cells to necrosis mediated by tumor necrosis factor. *Journal of Experimental Medicine*, *187*, 1477−1485.

Vorobjeva, N. V., & Pinegin, B. V. (2014). Neutrophil extracellular traps: Mechanisms of formation and role in health and disease. *Biochemistry (Moscow)*, *79*, 1286−1296.

Wang, Y., Li, M., Stadler, S., Correll, S., Li, P., Wang, D., . . . Coonrod, S. A. (2009). Histone hypercitrullination mediates chromatin decondensation and neutrophil extracellular trap formation. *Journal of Cell Biology*, *184*, 205−213.

Warnatsch, A., Ioannou, M., Wang, Q., & Papayannopoulos, V. (2015). Neutrophil extracellular traps license macrophages for cytokine production in atherosclerosis. *Science*, *349*, 316−320.

Welin, A., Amirbeagi, F., Christenson, K., Björkman, L., Björnsdottir, H., & Forsman, H. (2013). The human neutrophil subsets defined by the presence or absence of OLFM4 both transmigrate into tissue in vivo and give rise to distinct NETs in vitro. *PLoS One*, *8*, e69575.

Xu, J. C., Fan, J., Wang, X., Eacker, S. M., Kam, Ti, Chen, L., . . . Dawson, V. L. (2016). Cultured networks of excitatory projection neurons and inhibitory interneurons for studying human cortical neurotoxicity. *Science Translational Medicine*, *8*, 333−348.

Yang, C. W., Strong, B. S. I., Miller, M. J., & Unanue, E. R. (2010). Neutrophils influence the level of antigen presentation during the immune response to protein antigens in adjuvants. *Journal of Immunology.*, *185*, 2927−2934.

Yoshida, M., Sasaki, M., Sugisaki, K., Yamaguchi, Y., & Yamada, M. (2013). Neutrophil extracellular trap components in fibrinoid necrosis of the kidney with myeloperoxidase-ANCA-associated vasculitis. *Clinical Kidney Journal.*, *6*, 308−312.

Yousefi, S., & Simon, H. U. (2009). Autophagy in cells of the blood. *Biochimica et Biophysica Acta*, *1793*, 1461−1464.

Zanetti, M. (2004). Cathelicidins, multifunctional peptides of the innate immunity. *Journal of Leukocyte Biology*, *75*, 39−48.

Zhai, R., Ge, X., Li, H., Tang, Z., Liao, R., & Kleinjans, J. (2004). Differences in cellular and inflammatory cytokine profiles in the bronchoalveolar lavage fluid in bagassosis and silicosis. *American Journal of Industrial Medicine, 46,* 338−344.

Further reading

Borges, V. M., Lopes, M. F., Falčao, H., Leite-Junior, J. H., Rocco, P. R., Davidson, W. F., . . . DosReis, G. A. (2002). Apoptosis underlies immunopathogenic mechanisms in acute silicosis. *American Journal of Respiratory Cell and Molecular Biology, 27,* 78−84.

Cao, S., Liu, P., Zhu, H., Gong, H., Yao, J., & Sun, Y. (2015). Extracellular Acidification Acts as a Key Modulator of Neutrophil Apoptosis and Functions. *PLoS One., 10,* 1−15.

Liu, Y., Wang, X., Jia, Y., & Liu, Y. (2017). Effects of bufalin on the mTOR/p70S6K pathway and apoptosis in esophageal squamous cell carcinoma in nude mice. *International Journal of Molecular Medicine, 40*(2), 357−366.

Liz, R., Simard, J. C., Leonardi, L. B. A., & Girard, D. (2015). Silver nanoparticles rapidly induce atypical human neutrophil cell death by a process involving inflammatory caspases and reactive oxygen species and induce neutrophil extracellular traps release upon cell adhesion. *International Immunopharmacology., 28,* 616−625.

Segawa, K., Suzuki, J., & Nagata, S. (2011). Constitutive exposure of phosphatidylserine on viable cells. *Proceedings of the National Academy of Sciences of the United States of America, 108,* 19246−19251.

Chapter 4

NETosis in neonates

Following encounter with foreign threats like microbial invasion, neutrophils are the primary leukocytes that reach the site of inflammation to execute their function of phagocytosing microbes and eventually killing them (Kolaczkowska & Kubes, 2013). In addition to this, neutrophils employ two more approaches to combat pathogens: degranulation, that is release of effective proteases and molecules from their granules, and neutrophil extracellular trap (NET) formation, that is formation of weblike structure to trap and kill the pathogens (Kolaczkowska & Kubes, 2013). Brinkmann et al. (2004) who first reported NET activity revealed that NET can be induced by interleukin 8 (IL-8), phorbol 12 mystrate 13 acetate (PMA), and lipopolysaccharide (LPS). As seen through scanning and confocal electron microscopy and further validated by proteomic analysis, NETs structure is armed with chromatin threads (DNA and histones) along with various antimicrobial peptides—neutrophil elastase (NE), myeloperoxidase (MPO) proteinase 3, cathepsin G, bactericidal/permeability-increasing protein (BPI), defensins, and cathelicidin (LL-37) (Brinkmann et al., 2004). NET formation can induce tissue damage along with entrapping pathogens. Interestingly, NET has both beneficial and detrimental effect in tissue.

NET formation is a unique defensive mechanism of polymorphonuclear neutrophils (PMNs) that allows them to capture, immobilize, and eventually kill microbes in the extracellular space (Brinkmann et al., 2004; Brinkmann & Zychlinsky, 2012; Sørensen & Borregaard, 2016). NET formation occurs by a novel cell death process often called NETosis, although "vital" NETosis, in which the neutrophils do not immediately die, has also been described (Yipp & Kubes, 2013; Yipp et al., 2012). The molecular mechanisms leading to NET formation are not completely understood and possibly depend on stimulus type (Brinkmann et al., 2004; Papayannopoulos, Metzler, Hakkim, & Zychlinsky, 2010; Sørensen & Borregaard, 2016; Yipp et al., 2012). However, decondensation of chromatin and extrusion of DNA together with histones and granule contents are major events (Brinkmann & Zychlinsky, 2012; Papayannopoulos et al., 2010; Sørensen & Borregaard, 2016; Yipp & Kubes, 2013; Yipp et al., 2012). Peptidyl arginine deiminase 4 (PAD4)−mediated deamination of histones is (Kolaczkowska et al., 2015; Li et al., 2010; Wang et al., 2009) thought to be a prerequisite for nuclear

NETosis. DOI: https://doi.org/10.1016/B978-0-12-816147-0.00004-6

decondensation and NET formation. NET-facilitated trapping and elimination of pathogens perhaps complement conventional PMN antimicrobial activities including phagocytosis and intracellular killing (Brinkmann & Zychlinsky, 2012).

Clinical observations clearly indicate that inefficient NET formation contributes to intractable infections in some occurrences (Bianchi et al., 2009; Brinkmann & Zychlinsky, 2012), but the prominence of NETs in pathogen killing in vivo remains unclear and debatable (Brinkmann & Zychlinsky, 2012; Sørensen & Borregaard, 2016; Yipp & Kubes, 2013). Experimental models and some clinical studies indicate that intra- or extravascular NET formation contributes to tissue injury in bacteremia (Clark et al., 2007; Kolaczkowska, et al., 2015; McDonald, Urrutia, Yipp, Jenne, & Kubes, 2012), transfusion-related acute lung injury (Caudrillier et al., 2012; Sayah et al., 2015), primary graft dysfunction after lung transplantation (Sayah et al., 2015), sterile vasculopathies and immune inflammation (Chen et al., 2014; Lood et al., 2016), thrombosis (Fuchs et al., 2010; Pillai et al., 2016). Thus NET formation may be an important ill-adjusted and unresolved activity of neutrophils (Sørensen & Borregaard, 2016) subject to inappropriate triggering or being unregulated in infection and inflammation.

Neutrophil activity during pregnancy and in newborns

During pregnancy, immune system plays a balancing role to protect both the mother and the fetus without affecting the development of the fetus (Mor, Cardenas, Abrahams, & Guller, 2011). Pregnancy is the most crucial condition where mother and fetus calmly cooperate to shield the fetus from immunological recognition and rejection. The period of pregnancy is characterized by immunomodulatory changes involved in every phase of pregnancy, along with the interaction with pathogens. In addition, pregnancy comprises proinflammatory phase during the first trimester, the antiinflammatory phase during the second trimester, and return to proinflammatory phase again at the end of pregnancy (Mor & Cardenas, 2010). It has been observed that pregnant women have highest number of leukocytes during the course of pregnancy, of which neutrophils are present in maximum numbers (Crocker, Baker, & Fletcher, 2000). However, these neutrophils have reduced respiratory burst at the time of second and third trimesters and their activity returns to normal within 7-week postpartum. Elevated amounts of cell-free DNA (cfDNA) (nucleosome/MPO complexes) are present in pregnant women's serum as compared to nonpregnant women (Sur Chowdhury et al., 2016). Formation of nucleosome/MPO complexes increases in pregnancy with preeclampsia as compared to women with normal pregnancy (Sur Chowdhury et al., 2016) as highest serum cfDNA level is observed in women with preeclampsia. Interestingly, it has been found that circulating plasma DNA of both fetal and maternal from preeclampsia women is proportional to the degree of disease severity (Zhong et al., 2001). Fetus has the capability to develop their own immune system in the uterus (Dauby, Goetghebuer, Kollmann, Levy, & Marchant, 2012). Immediately after birth both term and preterm newborns have reduced number of immune cells, which is observed to be augmented in the initial weeks of their life (Nguyen et al., 2016; Walker et al., 2011). Neutrophils start to form in the clavicular marrow after $11-12$ weeks of conception which grows to maximum numbers after $13-15$ weeks (Slayton, Juul, et al., 1998; Slayton, Li, et al., 1998). Neutrophils are the most abundant immune cells in newborns as neuropoiesis starts in fetal liver and yolk sac during fifth week (Kolaczkowska & Kubes, 2013; Sperandio et al., 2013). In adults, neutrophils are capable of migrating to the site of infection and effectively fight against pathogens by phagocytosis or degranulations (Bektas, Goetze, & Speer, 1990; Nupponen et al., 2002). Term neonates are equally efficient in accomplishing degranulations and phagocytosis like adults. However, both these neutrophils' functions are found to be impaired in preterm neonates. It has been reported by McEvoy, Zakem-Cloud, and Tosi (1996) and Nussbaum et al. (2013) that both term and preterm neutrophils have impaired capability of migration to the site of inflammation and infection. Inefficient neutrophil activity makes neonates more susceptible to life-threatening infections and sepsis resulting in high morbidity and mortality rate (Gardner, 2009; Lawn, Kerber, Enweronu-Laryea, & Cousens, 2010). Reduced expression of surface adhesion molecules, and more number of immature neutrophils are also observed in newborns (Carr, Pumford, & Davies, 1992; Makoni, Eckert, Anne Pereira, Nizet, & Lawrence, 2016).

Human neonates have a common multifactorial syndrome of neutrophil dysfunction that is incompletely characterized and contributes to sepsis and other severe infectious complications. It has been noticed that human newborns are highly susceptible to sepsis and other life-threatening infections. The incidence and rate of infection are further higher in the low birth weight (LBW) newborns (<2.5 kg). Singh et al. (2013) compared the gene expressions and found that more than 1000 genes were downregulated in LBW newborns, of which most of them were associated with immune response and neutrophil function in particular (Fig. 4.1). The complete datasets compiling raw and normalized data from this study are available in the Gene Expression Omnibus repository (GEO series accession number: GSE29807). Disability in neutrophil functions may serve as one of the possible reason for this compromised immune activity in newborns.

Impaired and delayed NETosis in newborns

Human neonates have distinctive and complex immune regulation, marked by increased vulnerability toward infection and inflammatory pathology. The infant is in a protected and sterile environment in utero, but it can

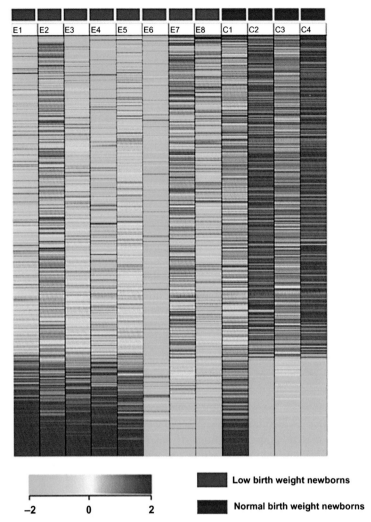

FIGURE 4.1 Expression profile of differentially expressed genes in low birth weight (LBW) newborns. The heat map illustrates the differences in gene expression profiles in the LBW newborns compared to NBW newborns groups where the columns E1−E8 correspond to LBW samples and C1−C4 correspond to NBW newborns samples.

encounter pathogens before or during labor (McDonagh et al., 2004). Newborns get colonized with bacteria soon after delivery, a process associated with increase in circulating and bone marrow neutrophils (Deshmukh et al., 2014; Jost, Lacroix, Braegger, & Chassard, 2012; McDonagh et al., 2004; Palmer, Bik, DiGiulio, Relman, & Brown, 2007). Such adaptations seem to have evolved to prevent extreme, injurious inflammation in the perinatal period and during sudden neonatal transition from the protected intrauterine environment to continuous microbial exposure (Dowling & Levy, 2014; Elahi et al., 2013). Interestingly, these adaptations may, however, lead to increased susceptibility to infection. Earlier it has been reported that the inability of PMNs isolated from umbilical cord blood of preterm and term infants to form NETs when stimulated was earlier reported by Yost et al. (2009) who also documented defect in their NET-mediated bacterial killing, suggesting such an adaptation. They reported that neutrophils from term and preterm neonates are unable to form NETs when stimulated by different agonists such as LPS, PAF, and fMLP. They have also noticed that these neonates have inefficient extracellular bacterial killing in addition to the NET formation. Reactive oxygen species (ROS) generation is also affected in newborns contributing to inefficient neutrophil activity. However, subsequent studies by other investigators showed that NET formation is temporarily delayed in newborns when their neutrophils were stimulated in vitro (Marcos et al., 2009). Lipp et al. (2017) reported that neutrophils from term infants generate NETs in stimulation with PMA, but preterm newborns show significantly lower NET structure. Inefficient NET formation may be an important aspect of immunodeficiency that inclines newborn infants resulting in infection.

Distinct neutrophil extracellular trap regulation exists in newborns

Although earlier reports suggested that NET formation is regulated via nicotinamide adenine dinucleotide phosphate (NADPH) oxidase enzyme by generating ROS, the deficiency in NET formation cannot be complimented by ROS donor (glucose oxidase) in preterm and term neonates as in case of adults. Byrd et al. (2016) showed that fibronectin (Fn) together with *Candida albicans* hyphae or Fn along with purified fungal β-glucan are able to form ROS-independent NETs in newborns. It seems neutrophils in newborns are more sensitive to fungal stimulation than to bacterial components. Marcos et al. (2009) also showed that neonatal neutrophils are able to form NETs upon LPS stimulation along with stimulation with several other TLR ligands Pam3CSK4, heat-killed *Listeria monocytogenes*, FSL-1, LPS, flagellin, ssRNA40, or ODN2006. It is evident from above studies that newborn's neutrophils exhibit delayed NET formation, as they take longer time for generating maximal NET. Interestingly, studies revealed that preterm infants gain the capacity to release NET by day 3 of birth and between day 3 and 14 of their life the maximum level of NET formation is achieved (Yost et al., 2016). Interestingly, in mammals like pigs NETs also exhibit similar features (Nguyen et al., 2016). Additionally, poor NET formation was observed in 21-day-old mice as compared to 60-day-old mice (Barth et al., 2016).

Calprotectin is associated with neutrophil extracellular trap in newborns

Calprotectin, an antibacterial protein present in neutrophils, is associated with activated macrophages in bowel (Gordon, Swanson, Clark, & Spitzer, 2015; Maheshwari et al., 2014). Presence of calprotectin is also observed in monocytes and macrophages. It accounts for 60% of all cytosolic proteins (Alibrahim, Aljasser, & Salh, 2015; Bin-Nun et al., 2015; Menees, Powell, Kurlander, Goel, & Chey, 2015). Calprotectin stabilizes and prevents degradation of calcium by binding with it (Waugh et al., 2013). Migration of activated neutrophils through gastrointestinal epithelial membrane causes high levels of calprotectin in stool (Wright, De Cruz, Gearry, Day, & Kamm, 2014). It has been reported that newborns suffering from necrotizing enterocolitis (NEC) have higher levels of calprotectin in their stool than healthy neonates (Bin-Nun et al., 2015; Carroll, Corfield, Spicer, & Cairns, 2003). Reports suggest that calprotectin is one of the major proteins released by neutrophils in association with NETs in expurgated NEC-affected bowel. Therefore presence of neutrophil-derived calprotectin to some extent, in stools of newborns suffering with NEC, migrates to the intestinal mucosa and lumen and further induces antimicrobial calprotectin from NETosis (MacQueen et al., 2016).

Inhibitors of neutrophil extracellular trap activity in newborns

Yost et al. (2016) reported a family of endogenous inhibitors of NETs in neonates responsible for impaired/delayed NET formation in them. The first identified peptide being neonatal NET-inhibitory factor (nNIF), they called this family of inhibitors as nNIF-related peptides (NRPs). NRPs also constitute cancer-associated structuredness of the cytoplasmic matrix (SCM) recognition, immune defense suppression and serine protease protection peptide (CRISPP) and a 44 amino acid carboxy terminus cleavage fragment of A1AT (α1-antitrypsin), A1ATm358. Variation in NETs between preterm and term newborns is reported. The reason behind this can be that inhibitors described above decrease quickly in the newborns after delivery. This can be a possible reason for differential NET formation between term and preterm infants. The inhibitors were also detected in different tissues/body fluids such as placenta (A1ATm358), umbilical blood (nNIF), and plasma (CRISPP-related peptides), which clearly emphasizes their utility in newborns. They are able to prevent NET formation stimulated by PMA, damage-associated molecular pattern (heme), and with live bacteria (*Staphylococcus aureus*), however, they are unable to neutralize them (Yost et al., 2016). A fascinating phenomenon associated with NRPs is they do not alter ROS production. Interestingly, NRPs neither affect ROS production nor affect NE activity; however, they are able to restrict PAD4-mediated histone citrullination. In addition to this, the injection of either nNIF or CRISPP into adult mice infected with *Escherichia coli* or LPS prevented formation of NETs and decreased bacterial killing (Yost et al., 2016).

Interestingly, it has been observed that in contrast to newborns nNIF is present in almost negligible amount in healthy adults and at untraceable levels in plasma of adults having chronic inflammatory disorders (Yost et al., 2016). The possible reason behind lower levels of nNIF in adults could be the generation of NET stimuli at the maternal−fetal boundary (Gupta, Hasler, Holzgreve, Gebhardt, & Hahn, 2005; Marder et al., 2016; Mizugishi & Yamashita, 2017), and to avoid excessive formation of the traps that could cause inflammatory pathology in the feto-maternal interface nNIF may be needed, whereas in adults this scenario is irrelevant. However, after birth how the inhibitors are degraded or neutralized is not yet known.

Reactive oxygen species-independent pathway in newborns

ROS generation is an integral part of NET formation. However, in response to fungal β-glucan, neonatal neutrophils have been shown to release NET in an ROS-independent manner. Purified β-glucan and *C. albicans* hyphae in the context of fibronectin are capable of producing NETs. Isolated from fungal cell wall, purified β-glucan is able to mimic the effect of intact hyphae upon activation of neutrophils, which proves the effectiveness of this cell wall component in innate immune response. Large *C. albicans* hyphae are too tough to be ingested by phagocytosis; therefore, to combat with fungal infections, neutrophils operate via mechanism that does not involve internalization. In this context, in the absence of phagocytosis immobilization of β-glucan thereby works as a reductionist model of neutrophil receptiveness to this key fungal PAMP. In adults, the β2 integrin CR3 present on the neutrophil surface was essential for NET release and aggregation (Byrd et al., 2016). According to Yost et al. (2009), neutrophils from premature and healthy term infants were shown to be impaired in forming adequate amount of NETs when challenged with inflammatory agonists such as PMA, PAF, and LPS. Byrd et al. (2016) suggested that neonatal PMNs formed minimal NETs to inflammatory agonists confirming results by Yost et al. (2009). They have shown robust aggregation and NETosis of neonatal PMNs in response to Fn with β-glucan. It has been reported that NET killing of *C. albicans* by adult neutrophils was ROS independent and confirmed that neutrophils maintained their fungicidal activity when infected with immobilized Fn with β-glucan. Report suggests that in neonates oxidative burst and NET release are uncoupled phenomena during the response to fungal PAMP β-glucan or intact *C. albicans* hyphae (Byrd et al., 2016).

Differential regulation of neutrophil extracellular traps components in newborns

NET formation has been found to be impaired in cord neutrophils (Yost et al., 2009). Zhu et al. (2014) reported 24 proteins involved in NETs (Guimaraes-Costa, Nascimento, Wardini, Pinto-da-Silva, & Saraiva, 2012). Interestingly, some of these proteins were expressed at differential levels in cord and adult neutrophils. Only one protein was upregulated and the six were downregulated in cord neutrophils. Seventeen proteins that expressed at similar levels were mostly NET components and included histones and granule proteins, cytosolic and cytoskeleton proteins, catalase and glycolytic enzymes. These similarly expressed proteins were characterized for biological function using STRING tool and were found to regulate several functional clusters some of which were *the apoptosis-related protein cluster*, including catalase, alpha-actinin-1, S100 calcium-binding protein A9 (S1009A), and mycloid ccll nuclcar differentiation antigen; the *cytoskeleton clusters* comprising of myosin-9 (MYH9), plastin-2 (LCP1), alpha-actinin-1, and S1009A. Six proteins, cathepsin G, BPI, S1008A, S1009A, S10012A, and lactoferroxin-C were involved in the function of *response to bacteria*. It was reported that six proteins were underexpressed in cord neutrophils. Proteins that were underexpressed in newborns' cord blood−derived neutrophils included three that were major components of azurophilic granule, the specialized lysosomes for killing microorganisms in neutrophils, NE is known as an ELANE expressed specifically in neutrophils. It plays key roles in NETosis and inhibition of its activity eliminated NET formation, MPO produces hypohalous acids central to the microbicidal activity of neutrophils and also triggers ELANE to promote nuclear decondensation and NETosis (Papayannopoulos et al., 2010) and the third one azurocidin (AZU1) has antibiotic activity and also acts as a multifunctional inflammatory mediator or a potent chemoattractant to monocytes, lymphocytes and, to some extent, neutrophils (Chertov et al., 1997). The downregulation of these major components of azurophilic granule in cord neutrophils leads to impaired NETosis in the immature neutrophils. Matrix metalloproteases (MMPs) or endopeptidases are the key proteases involved in extracellular matrix degradation. In addition to this, MMPs have crucial roles in neutrophil migration (Elkington, O'Kane, & Friedland, 2005). MMP9 is stored in neutrophil-specific granules, being robustly released after cellular activation and implicated in extracellular matrix remodeling and cell migration during acute inflammation (Warner et al., 2001). Its remarkable downregulation in cord neutrophils clearly implicates its crucial roles not only in the NETosis, but also in impaired transmigration under stress condition.

References

Alibrahim, B., Aljasser, M. I., & Salh, B. (2015). Fecal calprotectin use in inflammatory bowel disease and beyond: A mini-review. *Canadian Journal of Gastroenterology & Hepatology*, *29*(3), 157–163.

Barth, C. R., Luft, C., Funchal, G. A., de Oliveira, J. R., Porto, B. N., & Donadio, M. V. F. (2016). LPS-induced neonatal stress in mice affects the response profile to an inflammatory stimulus in an age and sex-dependent manner. *Developmental Psychobiology*, *58*(5), 600–613. Available from https://doi.org/10.1002/dev.21404.

Bektas, S., Goetze, B., & Speer, C. P. (1990). Decreased adherence, chemotaxis and phagocytic activities of neutrophils from preterm neonates. *Acta Paediatrica Scandinavica*, *79*(11), 1031–1038.

Bianchi, M., Hakkim, A., Brinkmann, V., Siler, U., Seger, R. A., Zychlinsky, A., & Reichenbach, J. (2009). Restoration of NET formation by gene therapy in CGD controls aspergillosis. *Blood*, *114*(13), 2619–2622. Available from https://doi.org/10.1182/blood-2009-05-221606.

Bin-Nun, A., Booms, C., Sabag, N., Mevorach, R., Algur, N., & Hammerman, C. (2015). Rapid fecal calprotectin (FC) analysis: Point of care testing for diagnosing early necrotizing enterocolitis. *American Journal of Perinatology*, *32*(4), 337–342. Available from https://doi.org/10.1055/s-0034-1384640.

Brinkmann, V., Reichard, U., Goosmann, C., Fauler, B., Uhlemann, Y., Weiss, D. S., ... Zychlinsky, A. (2004). Neutrophil extracellular traps kill bacteria. *Science*, *303*(5663), 1532–1535.

Brinkmann, V., & Zychlinsky, A. (2012). Neutrophil extracellular traps: Is immunity the second function of chromatin? *The Journal of Cell Biology*, *198*(5), 773–783.

Byrd, A. S., O'Brien, X. M., Laforce-Nesbitt, S. S., Parisi, V. E., Hirakawa, M. P., Bliss, J. M., & Reichner, J. S. (2016). NETosis in neonates: Evidence of a reactive oxygen species-independent pathway in response to fungal challenge. *The Journal of Infectious Diseases*, *213*(4), 634–639.

Carr, R., Pumford, D., & Davies, J. M. (1992). Neutrophil chemotaxis and adhesion in preterm babies. *Archives of Disease in Childhood*, *67*(7 Spec No), 813–817.

Carroll, D., Corfield, A., Spicer, R., & Cairns, P. (2003). Faecal calprotectin concentrations and diagnosis of necrotising enterocolitis. *Lancet*, *361*(9354), 310–311.

Caudrillier, A., Kessenbrock, K., Gilliss, B. M., Nguyen, J. X., Marques, M. B., Monestier, M., ... Looney, M. R. (2012). Platelets induce neutrophil extracellular traps in transfusion-related acute lung injury. *The Journal of Clinical Investigation*, *122*(7), 2661–2671.

Chen, G., Zhang, D., Fuchs, T. A., Manwani, D., Wagner, D. D., & Frenette, P. S. (2014). Heme-induced neutrophil extracellular traps contribute to the pathogenesis of sickle cell disease. *Blood*, *123*(24), 3818–3827.

Chertov, O., Ueda, H., Xu, L. L., Tani, K., Murphy, W. J., Wang, J. M., ... Oppenheim, J. J. (1997). Identification of human neutrophil-derived cathepsin G and azurocidin/CAP37 as chemoattractants for mononuclear cells and neutrophils. *The Journal of Experimental Medicine*, *186*(5), 739–747.

Clark, S. R., Ma, A. C., Tavener, S. A., McDonald, B., Goodarzi, Z., Kelly, M. M., ... Kubes, P. (2007). Platelet TLR4 activates neutrophil extracellular traps to ensnare bacteria in septic blood. *Nature Medicine*, *13*(4), 463–469.

Crocker, I. P., Baker, P. N., & Fletcher, J. (2000). Neutrophil function in pregnancy and rheumatoid arthritis. *Annals of the Rheumatic Diseases*, *59*(7), 555–564.

Dauby, N., Goetghebuer, T., Kollmann, T. R., Levy, J., & Marchant, A. (2012). Uninfected but not unaffected: Chronic maternal infections during pregnancy, fetal immunity, and susceptibility to postnatal infections. *The Lancet. Infectious Diseases, 12*(4), 330−340.

Deshmukh, H. S., Liu, Y., Menkiti, O. R., Mei, J., Dai, N., O'Leary, C. E., ... Worthen, G. S. (2014). The microbiota regulates neutrophil homeostasis and host resistance to *Escherichia coli* K1 sepsis in neonatal mice. *Nature Medicine, 20*(5), 524−530.

Dowling, D. J., & Levy, O. (2014). Ontogeny of early life immunity. *Trends in Immunology, 35* (7), 299−310.

Elahi, S., Ertelt, J. M., Kinder, J. M., Jiang, T. T., Zhang, X., Xin, L., ... Way, S. S. (2013). Immunosuppressive CD71 + erythroid cells compromise neonatal host defence against infection. *Nature, 504*(7478), 158−162.

Elkington, P. T., O'Kane, C. M., & Friedland, J. S. (2005). The paradox of matrix metalloproteinases in infectious disease. *Clinical and Experimental Immunology, 142*(1), 12−20.

Fuchs, T. A., Brill, A., Duerschmied, D., Schatzberg, D., Monestier, M., Myers, D. D., Jr., ... Wagner, D. D. (2010). Extracellular DNA traps promote thrombosis. *Proceedings of the National Academy of Sciences of the United States of America, 107*(36), 15880−15885.

Gardner, S. L. (2009). Sepsis in the neonate. *Critical Care Nursing Clinics of North America, 21* (1), 121−141.

Gordon, P. V., Swanson, J. R., Clark, R., & Spitzer, A. (2015). The complete blood cell count in a refined cohort of preterm NEC: The importance of gestational age and day of diagnosis when using the CDC to estimate mortality. *Journal of Perinatology: Official Journal of the California Perinatal Association, 36*(2), 121−125.

Guimaraes-Costa, A. B., Nascimento, M. T., Wardini, A. B., Pinto-da-Silva, L. H., & Saraiva, E. M. (2012). ETosis: A microbicidal mechanism beyond cell death. *Journal of Parasitology Research, 929743.* Available from https://doi.org/10.1155/2012/929743.

Gupta, A. K., Hasler, P., Holzgreve, W., Gebhardt, S., & Hahn, S. (2005). Induction of neutrophil extracellular DNA lattices by placental microparticles and IL-8 and their presence in preeclampsia. *Human Immunology, 66*(11), 1146−1154.

Jost, T., Lacroix, C., Braegger, C. P., & Chassard, C. (2012). New insights in gut microbiota establishment in healthy breast fed neonates. *PLoS One, 7*(8), e44595. Available from https://doi.org/10.1371/journal.pone.0044595.

Kolaczkowska, E., Jenne, C. N., Surewaard, B. G., Thanabalasuriar, A., Lee, W. Y., Sanz, M. J., ... Kubes, P. (2015). Molecular mechanisms of NET formation and degradation revealed by intravital imaging in the liver vasculature. *Nature Communications, 6,* 6673. Available from https://doi.org/10.1038/ncomms7673.

Kolaczkowska, E., & Kubes, P. (2013). Neutrophil recruitment and function in health and inflammation. *Nature Reviews. Immunology, 13*(3), 159−175.

Lawn, J. E., Kerber, K., Enweronu-Laryea, C., & Cousens, S. (2010). 3.6 million neonatal deaths—What is progressing and what is not? *Seminar Perinatology, 34*(6), 371−386.

Li, P., Li, M., Lindberg, M. R., Kennett, M. J., Xiong, N., & Wang, Y. (2010). PAD4 is essential for antibacterial innate immunity mediated by neutrophil extracellular traps. *Journal of Experimental Medicine, 207*(9), 1853−1862.

Lipp, P., Ruhnau, J., Lange, A., Vogelgesang, A., Dressel, A., & Heckmann, M. (2017). Less neutrophil extracellular trap formation in term newborns than in adults. *Neonatology, 111* (2), 182−188.

Lood, C., Blanco, L. P., Purmalek, M. M., Carmona-Rivera, C., De Ravin, S. S., Smith, C. K., ... Kaplan, M. J. (2016). Neutrophil extracellular traps enriched in oxidized mitochondrial

DNA are interferogenic and contribute to lupus-like disease. *Nature Medicine*, *22*(2), 146−153.

MacQueen, B. C., Christensen, R. D., Yost, C. C., Lambert, D. K., Baer, V. L., Sheffield, M. J., . . . Shepherd, J. G. (2016). Elevated fecal calprotectin levels during necrotizing enterocolitis are associated with activated neutrophils extruding neutrophil extracellular. *Journal of Perinatology: Official Journal of the California Perinatal Association*, *36*(10), 862−869.

Maheshwari, A., Schelonka, R. L., Dimmitt, R. A., Carlo, W. A., Munoz-Hernandez, B., Das, A., . . . Higgins, R. D. (2014). Cytokines associated with necrotizing enterocolitis in extremely-low-birth-weight infants. *Pediatric Research*, *76*(1), 100−108.

Makoni, M., Eckert, J., Anne Pereira, H., Nizet, V., & Lawrence, S. M. (2016). Alterations in neonatal neutrophil function attributable to increased immature forms. *Early Human Development*, *103*, 1−7. Available from https://doi.org/10.1016/j.earlhumdev.2016.05.016.

Marcos, V., Nussbaum, C., Vitkov, L., Hector, A., Wiedenbauer, E. M., Roos, D., . . . Hartl, D. (2009). Delayed but functional neutrophil extracellular trap formation in neonates. *Blood*, *114*(23), 4908−4911.

Marder, W., Knight, J. S., Kaplan, M. J., Somers, E. C., Zhang, X., O'Dell, A. A., . . . Lieberman, R. W. (2016). Placental histology and neutrophil extracellular traps in lupus and pre-eclampsia pregnancies. *Lupus Science and Medicine*, *3*(1), e000134. Available from https://doi.org/10.1136/lupus-2015-000134.

McDonagh, S., Maidji, E., Ma, W., Chang, H. T., Fisher, S., & Pereira, L. (2004). Viral and bacterial pathogens at the maternal-fetal interface. *Journal of Infectious Diseases*, *190*(4), 826−834.

McDonald, B., Urrutia, R., Yipp, B. G., Jenne, C. N., & Kubes, P. (2012). Intravascular neutrophil extracellular traps capture bacteria from the bloodstream during sepsis. *Cell Host & Microbe*, *12*(3), 324−333.

McEvoy, L. T., Zakem-Cloud, H., & Tosi, M. F. (1996). Total cell content ofCR3 (CD11b/CD18) and LFA-1 (CD11a/CD18) in neonatal neutrophils: Relationship to gestational age. *Blood*, *87*(9), 3929−3933.

Menees, S. B., Powell, C., Kurlander, J., Goel, A., & Chey, W. D. (2015). A meta-analysis of the utility of C-reactive protein, erythrocyte sedimentation rate, fecal calprotectin, and fecal lactoferrin to exclude inflammatory bowel disease in adults with IBS. *The American Journal of Gastroenterology*, *110*(3), 444−454.

Mizugishi, K., & Yamashita, K. (2017). Neutrophil extracellular traps are critical for pregnancy loss in sphingosine kinase−deficient mice on 129Sv/C57BL/6 background. *The Federation of American Societies for Experimental Biology Journal*, *31*(12), 5577−5591. Available from https://doi.org/10.1096/fj.201700399RR.

Mor, G., & Cardenas, I. (2010). The immune system in pregnancy: A unique complexity. *American Journal of Reproductive Immunology*, *63*(6), 425−433.

Mor, G., Cardenas, I., Abrahams, V., & Guller, S. (2011). Inflammation and pregnancy: The role of the immune system at the implantation site. *Annals of the New York Academy of Sciences*, *1221*, 80−87. Available from https://doi.org/10.1111/j.1749-6632.2010.05938.x.

Nguyen, D. N., Jiang, P., Frøkiær, H., Heegaard, P. M. H., Thymann, T., & Sangild, P. T. (2016). Delayed development of systemic immunity in preterm pigs as a model for preterm infants. *Scientific Reports*, *6*, 36816. Available from https://doi.org/10.1038/srep36816.

Nupponen, I., Turunen, R., Nevalainen, T., Peuravuori, H., Pohjavuori, M., Repo, H., & Andersson, S. (2002). Extracellular release of bactericidal/permeability-increasing protein in newborn infants. *Pediatric Research*, *51*, 670−674.

Nussbaum, C., Gloning, A., Pruenster, M., Frommhold, D., Bierschenk, S., Genzel-Boroviczény, O., ... Sperandio, M. (2013). Neutrophil and endothelial adhesive function during human fetal ontogeny. *Journal of Leukocyte Biology*, *93*(2), 175−184.

Palmer, C., Bik, E. M., DiGiulio, D. B., Relman, D. A., & Brown, P. O. (2007). Development of the human infant intestinal microbiota. *PLoS Biology*, *5*(7), e177.

Papayannopoulos, V., Metzler, K. D., Hakkim, A., & Zychlinsky, A. (2010). Neutrophil elastase and myeloperoxidase regulate the formation of neutrophil extracellular traps. *Journal of Cell Biology*, *191*(3), 677−691.

Pillai, P. S., Molony, R. D., Martinod, K., Dong, H., Pang, I. K., Tal, M. C., ... Iwasaki, A. (2016). Mx1 reveals innate pathways to antiviral resistance and lethal influenza disease. *Science*, *2352*(6284), 463−466.

Sayah, D. M., Mallavia, B., Liu, F., Ortiz-Muñoz, G., Caudrillier, A., DerHovanessian, A., ... Ardehali, A. (2015). Neutrophil extracellular traps are pathogenic in primary graft dysfunction after lung transplantation. *American Journal of Respiratory and Critical Care Medicine*, *191*(4), 455−463.

Singh, V. V., Chauhan, S. K., Rai, R., Kumar, A., Singh, S. M., & Rai, G. (2013). Decreased pattern recognition receptor signaling, increasing protein gene expression in cord blood of term low birth weight human newborns. *PLoS One*, *8*(4), e62845. Available from https://doi. org/10.1371/journal.pone.0062845.

Slayton, W. B., Juul, S. E., Calhoun, D. A., Li, Y., Braylan, R. C., & Christensen, R. D. (1998). Hematopoiesis in the liver and marrow of human fetuses at 5 to 16 weeks postconception: Quantitative assessment of macrophage and neutrophil populations. *Pediatric Research*, *43* (6), 774−782.

Slayton, W. B., Li, Y., Calhoun, D. A., Juul, S. E., Iturraspe, J., Braylan, R. C., & Christensen, R. D. (1998). The first-appearance of neutrophils in the human fetal bone marrow cavity. *Early Human Development*, *53*(2), 129−144.

Sørensen, O. E., & Borregaard, N. (2016). Neutrophil extracellular traps − The dark side of neutrophils. *Journal of Clinical Investigation*, *126*(5), 1612−1620.

Sperandio, M., Quackenbush, E. J., Sushkova, N., Altstätter, J., Nussbaum, C., Schmid, S., ... von Andrian, U. H. (2013). Ontogenetic regulation of leukocyte recruitment in mouse yolk sac vessels. *Blood*, *121*(21), e118−e128. Available from https://doi.org/10.1182/blood-2012-07-447144.

Sur Chowdhury, C., Hahn, S., Hasler, P., Hoesli, I., Lapaire, O., & Giaglis, S. (2016). Elevated levels of total cell-free DNA in maternal serum samples arise from the generation of neutrophil extracellular traps. *Fetal Diagnosis and Therapy*, *40*(4), 263−267.

Walker, J. C., Smolders, M. A. J. C., Gemen, E. F. A., Antonius, T. A. J., Leuvenink, J., & de Vries, E. (2011). Development of lymphocyte subpopulations in preterm infants. *Scandinavian Journal of Immunology*, *73*(1), 53−58.

Wang, Y., Li, M., Stadler, S., Correll, S., Li, P., Wang, D., ... Coonrod, S. A. (2009). Histone hypercitrullination mediates chromatin decondensation and neutrophil extracellular trap formation. *Journal of Cell Biology*, *184*(2), 205−213.

Warner, R. L., Beltran, L., Younkin, E. M., Lewis, C. S., Weiss, S. J., Varani, J., & Johnson, K. J. (2001). Role of stromelysin 1 and gelatinase B in experimental acute lung injury. *American Journal of Respiratory Cell and Molecular Biology*, *24*(5), 537−544.

Waugh, N., Cummins, E., Royle, P., Kandala, N. B., Shyangdan, D., Arasaradnam, R., ... Johnston, R. (2013). Faecal calprotectin testing for differentiating amongst inflammatory and non-inflammatory bowel diseases: Systematic review and economic evaluation. *Health Technology Assessment*, *17*(55). Available from https://doi.org/10.3310/hta17550, pp. xv−xix, 1−211.

Wright, E. K., De Cruz, P., Gearry, R., Day, A. S., & Kamm, M. A. (2014). Fecal biomarkers in the diagnosis and monitoring of Crohn's disease. *Inflammatory Bowel Disease, 20*(9), 1668−1677.

Yipp, B. G., & Kubes, P. (2013). NETosis: How vital is it? *Blood, 122*(16), 2784−2794.

Yipp, B. G., Petri, B., Salina, D., Jenne, C. N., Scott, B. N., Zbytnuik, L. D., ... Kubes, P. (2012). Infection-induced NETosis is a dynamic process involving neutrophil multitasking in vivo. *Nature Medicine, 8*(9), 1386−1393.

Yost, C. C., Cody, M. J., Harris, E. S., Thornton, N. L., McInturff, A. M., Martinez, M. L., ... Zimmerman, G. A. (2009). Impaired neutrophil extracellular trap (NET) formation: A novel innate immune deficiency of human neonates. *Blood, 113*(25), 6419−6427.

Yost, C. C., Schwertz, H., Cody, M. J., Wallace, J. A., Campbell, R. A., Vieira-de-Abreu, A., ... Zimmerman, G. A. (2016). Neonatal NET-inhibitory factor and related peptides inhibit neutrophil extracellular trap formation. *Journal of Clinical Investigation, 126*(10), 3783−3798.

Zhong, X. Y., Laivuori, H., Livingston, J. C., Ylikorkala, O., Sibai, B. M., Holzgreve, W., & Hahn, S. (2001). Elevation of both maternal and fetal extracellular circulating deoxyribonucleic acid concentrations in the plasma of pregnant women with preeclampsia. *American Journal of Obstetrics and Gynecology, 184*(3), 414−419.

Zhu, J., Zhang, H., Guo, T., Li, W., Li, H., & Zhu, Y. (2014). Quantitative proteomics reveals differential biological processes in healthy neonatal cord neutrophils and adult neutrophils. *Proteomics, 14*(13−14), 1688−1697. Available from https://doi.org/10.1002/pmic. 201400009.

Chapter 5

NETosis in Autoimmunity

Autoimmunity is defined as an immune response resulting from host's own immune system attacks to the self-tissue due to the loss of body's self-tolerance ability. Self-reactivity can arise either through the activation of immune receptors directly by autoantigen or due to cross-reactivity between foreign and self-antigens. Autoimmune disease is a clinical condition that results from this dysfunction of the immune system which otherwise serves to protect you from disease and infection. Autoimmunity can contribute to an ongoing disease by heightening and extending the pathology. One of the proposed mechanisms for autoimmunity is through posttranslational modifications that promote generation of neo-(auto) antigens, mounting up an autoimmune response.

As discussed in earlier chapters NETosis is a novel antimicrobial mechanism employed by neutrophils for conferring protection to the host but dysregulated neutrophil extracellular trap (NET) formation can also stimulate autoimmunity by generating autoantibodies against various NET components. NETs are a major source of autoantigens in autoimmune diseases. It has been observed that autoantibodies from patients with autoimmunity target innate immune defense proteins, including major NET factors such as elastase, cathepsin G, and proteinase 3 (Manolova, Dancheva, & Halacheva, 2001; Pradhan, Badakere, Bichile, & Almeida, 2004; Tamiya et al., 2006) as well as bactericidal peptides stored in granules and copurify with NETs such as neutrophil defensins and the LL37 peptide (Froy and Sthoeger, 2009; Lande et al., 2011). Deiminated autoantigens are primary autoantigens generated from NETs and neutrophils from an autoimmune disease like rheumatoid arthritis (RA) are more susceptible to NETosis than neutrophils of osteoarthritis (Khandpur et al., 2013). NETs also lead to stimulation of inflammatory responses, including the elevated expression of adhesion molecules, cytokines, and chemokines (Khandpur et al., 2013). Reports have suggested increased profusion of activated neutrophils and upregulated concentrations of neutrophil granule components in the sera of patients with more progressive disease (Manolova et al., 2001; Khandpur et al., 2013). It has been reported that complications of lupus positively correlate with the titers of anti-NET autoantibodies (Hakkim et al., 2010). Autoantibodies bind NET-associated proteins in lupus, in addition to the histones and DNA and the NETs' structural scaffold. Recent studies reveal the presence of

NETosis. DOI: https://doi.org/10.1016/B978-0-12-816147-0.00005-8
103

anti-peptidyl arginine deiminases (PAD)4 autoantibodies with the enzymatic activation of the diminase (Darrah et al., 2013). In the extracellular surroundings, PAD4 activation induces citrullinations of fibronectin, fibrinogen, collagen, and other matrix proteins that have been linked with manifestations of connective tissue. First, in the collagen-induced arthritis model, inhibition of PAD4 by Cl-amidine improved quantifiable disease symptoms in arthritis models (Willis et al., 2011). In addition, Cl-amidine also reduces myeloperoxidase (MPO) and immune complex deposition in the kidneys of NZM mice and improved endothelial cell differentiation and vasorelaxation, and reduces the risk of arterial thrombosis (Knight et al., 2013). Inhibitor of PADs deiminase activity improves neurodegenerative symptoms in a mouse model of multiple sclerosis (MS) (Wei et al., 2013). In sepsis condition, interaction of platelets with neutrophils triggers the activation of Toll-like receptors (TLR) pathways resulting into rapid formation of NETs. NETs are also detected in the lungs and plasma of transfusion-related acute lung injury (TRALI) as well as in alveoli of mice with antibody-mediated TRALI. One of the studies concluded that NETs are responsible for disruption in the endothelial cells and leakage in capillaries of lung (Caudrillier et al., 2012; Thomas et al., 2012). Interestingly, it has been observed that administration of antibody against histones and DNase I protects mice from TRALI and treatment with antihistone H4 antibody lowers the mortality rate in mice sepsis model. NETosis leads to accumulation of autoantigens-triggering autoimmune response in circulation. Often it has been observed that antinuclear antibodies against NETosis markers MPO and PR3 are present in in vitro and animal models of chronic autoimmune diseases. In addition, levels of circulating NETs were also elevated in active autoimmune patients (Yu and Su, 2013). These findings clearly indicate that NETosis generates enormous autoantibody pool triggering autoimmune response and also plays crucial roles in autoimmune disease progression such as RA, systemic lupus erythematosus (SLE), and MS.

NETosis in rheumatoid arthritis

RA is a chronic systemic autoimmune disease mostly affecting females than males and predominantly observed in the elderly. RA mostly affects the lining of the synovial joints triggering off gradual disability, early death, and socioeconomic worries. The clinical implication of symmetrical joint involvement includes arthralgia, swelling, redness, and even limiting the range of motion.

Rheumatoid arthritis pathogenesis

According to the presence or absence of anticitrullinated protein antibodies (ACPAs), two major types of RA have been reported. Citrullination occurs by the calcium-dependent enzyme PAD. During posttranslational modification, positively charged arginine changes into polar citrulline PAD which catalyzes ACPAs, the most abundant autoantigens in RA patient which can be detected in approximately 67% of RA patients. It can serve as a useful diagnostic marker for patients with early, undifferentiated arthritis offering an indication of disease progression to RA (Bizzaro et al., 2013; Nishimura et al., 2007) The ACPA-positive subset of RA develops more antagonistic clinical phenotype as compared to ACPA-negative subset of RA (Malmström, Catrina, & Klareskog, 2017). It has been reported that ACPA-negative RA has distinct genetic association patterns (Padyukov et al., 2011) and differential responses of immune cells to citrullinated antigens (Schuerwegh et al., 2010) than that of ACPA-positive subset.

The etiology and pathology of RA can be separated into various stages: (1) triggering, (2) maturation, (3) targeting, and (4) fulminant stage, concomitant with hyperplastic synovium, cartilage damage, bone erosion, and systemic consequences.

The appearance of ACPA is now widely used to diagnose and predict RA due to its high specificity ($>97\%$) in clinical practice. The prime cause of ACPA generation in circulation is aberrant antibody response against citrullinated proteins, comprising vimentin, fibrin type-II collagen, fibronectin, Epstein-Barr Nuclear Antigen 1 (EBNA-1), α-enolase, along with histones, ACPA can be generated by both genetic and environmental factors. HLA-Dr, more accurately HLA-Dr1 and HLA-Dr4, also known as "shared epitopes" (SEs) are the primary genetic risk factors found in ACPA-positive RA patients (Raychaudhuri et al., 2012). Not only joints, lung exposure to noxious agents, including silica dust, nanosized silica, smoke, or nanomaterials, are able to induce mucosal TLRs that activate $Ca2^+$-mediated PADs, but also antigen-presenting cells (APCs), such as classical dendritic cells (DCs) and B cells. Therefore joints may not be the only place of trigger for autoimmunity in RA (Mohamed et al., 2012; Stolt et al., 2010; Too et al., 2016). Some pathogens such as Porphyromonas *gingivalis* infection are reported to lead to the production of citrullinated autoantigens and the ACPA in two ways, one by cleaving citrullinated proteins at arginine residues and producing autoantigens (Wegner et al., 2010) and the second way is via stimulating NET formation. Thus NETosis induction takes place by ACPAs and which in turn contributes in generation of ACPAs (Khandpur et al., 2013).

NETosis as a source of autoantigens in rheumatoid arthritis

Different inflammatory stimuli induce histone deimination, chromatin decondensation, and NET formation in neutrophils and also in eosinophils and in mast cells. The web like structure produced to entrap and kill consists of DNA, cationic granule proteins, and antimicrobial peptides and histones. These histone proteins get deiminated, and arginines are converted in citrullines. Although deamination is a normal process, it shows deleterious effect in case of RA conditions. This is because the citrullinated protein gets deposited in tissues of RA patients and acts as autoantigen to provoke the generation of autoantibodies against them. This indeed triggers the host immune response in a self-destructive manner. Although the physiological process of deimination is augmented in inflammatory conditions, it develops only in individuals having genetic predisposition to RA and make antibodies to deiminated proteins. These antibodies, known as ACPA, can interact with different deiminated proteins due to overlapping specificities. It has been observed that ACPA is the most abundant antibody in RA and owing to its high specificity and specificity they are used as diagnostic tool for RA characterization. The enormous genetic diversity in ACPA is due to somatic hypermutation in their variable Ig domains, which suggests that this is an antigen-driven response (Amara et al., 2013). Initially autoimmune responses to citrullinated proteins are impeded, but as the disease progresses the autoimmune response becomes prominent leading to increasing illness (Brink et al., 2013). The targets of ACPA include autoantigens (vimentin, fibrinogen, filaggrin, collagen II, and histones) as well as exogenous antigens (i.e., alpha-enolase, EBNA 1, and EBNA-2 proteins).

Citrullination or deimination, seen in RA, is catalyzed by the calcium-dependent enzyme PAD that makes these proteins susceptible for ACPA. PADs can be activated by Ca2 + influx from their inactive form as a result of different stimuli most likely ionophore-induced apoptosis of macrophages generating extracellular calcium influx (Asaga, Yamada, & Senshu, 1998) or lipopolysaccharide stimulation of neutrophils resulting into intracellular calcium mobilization. It has been well rooted that PAD activation by calcium influx generation in neutrophils is an apoptosis-independent route and occurs without caspase activation (Neeli, Khan, & Radic, 2008). PADs can be secreted from the cell and become activated, as a result of the extracellular Ca^{2+} concentration (Spengler et al., 2015). Citrullination is a natural physiological process that maintains the homeostasis of several organs but gets abruptly amplified during inflammation. In RA, multiple proteins are citrullinated, especially in target organs of the disease, mainly the synovium but also in the lungs (Lugli et al., 2015) and in myocardial tissue (Giles et al., 2012). Initially it has been suggested that fibrin is the most citrullinated protein in RA joints (Iobagiu et al., 2011), but now the presence of citrullinated vimentin and aggrecan is also detected (Glant et al., 2016). Citrullination plays a pathophysiological role in other inflammatory disorders other than RA such as the inflamed skeletal muscle tissue in myositis (Makrygiannakis et al., 2006) and the synovium of spondyloarthritis patients (Kinloch et al., 2008). A vast number of stimulants of neutrophils (cytokines, TLR ligands, etc.) can lead to generation of deiminated histones (Neeli et al., 2008). Perforin and complement membranolytic pathways enable pore formation in neutrophil membranes, which accelerates the intracellular calcium concentration and favoring the activity of PAD enzymes (Romero et al., 2013). Thus perforin and complement activation with membrane attack complex formation play an important role in the induction of abundant protein citrullination in synovial fluid neutrophils.

A significant contribution of these citrullinated proteins comes from the ability of RA neutrophils from peripheral blood or synovial fluid to form NETs. This process can be triggered by stimulants or it can happen spontaneously (Khandpur et al., 2013). Higher levels of deminitated H3 pools in RA patients as compared with controls were suggestive of higher spontaneous NETosis in their circulating neutrophils (Dwivedi et al., 2014). In addition to this, exposure to RA immunoglobulins or purified ACPA stimulates NET formation, and netting neutrophils have been detected in synovial tissue and rheumatoid nodules from RA patients (Khandpur et al., 2013). In synovial fluid, netting neutrophils secrete enzymatically active PAD2 and PAD4 in inflamed joints which may citrullinate extracellular proteins under local conditions. Presence of both soluble and NET-associated PAD suggests that NET acts as a molecular scaffold for protein citrullination (Spengler et al., 2015). Recent studies have described the mechanisms behind NET regulation by PAD4. Apart from ACPA, elevated level of MPO is found in RA patients. Studies in mouse model show that NADP oxidase, one of the prime mediator of NETosis, has some potential role in pathogenesis of RA (Jorch and Kubes, 2017).

In RA, a single nucleotide polymorphism (SNP) at position 1858 (C1858T) in the DNA encoding a protein tyrosine phosphatase (PTPN22), which results in the conversion of an arginine (R620) to a tryptophan (W620), has been identified (Begovich et al., 2004). Some SNPs have shown connection with disease progression with RA (Chang, Dwivedi, Nicholas, & Ho, 2015), although these SNPs are also detected in other autoimmune disease SLE, type I diabetes. In RA patients, NETs are able to activate synoviocytes, increase the production of proinflammatory cytokines, and amplify joint inflammation.

Thus neutrophils play an active role in the inflammatory process of RA serving as the source of and posttranslationally modified autoantigens (Mantovani, Cassatella, Costantini, & Jaillon, 2011).

Citrullination of histones in neutrophils in rheumatoid arthritis

The core nucleosome, comprising an H3—H4 tetramer and two H2A/H2B dimers, is not a static DNA packaging structure, but on the contrary is a dynamic complex, and the modulation of its structure is an important component of transcriptional regulation. Modifications in the conformation of histones, highly conserved in eukaryotic cells, from yeast to humans, are widely used in the dynamic modulation of chromatin structure and function. Twenty types of histone posttranslational modifications have been described, which are able to modulate chromatin function either by altering the amino acid charge and consequently the internucleosomal interactions or by enabling/inhibiting interactions with specific binding proteins external to nucleosomes but nonetheless essential for DNA regulation. Among all, one of the latest described is the deimination of arginine. The first description of histone deimination was reported by Hagiwara, Hidaka, and Yamada (2005). They observed that when HL60-derived granulocytes and peripheral blood granulocytes are stimulated with A23187 (a mobile ion-carrier known as calcium ionophore), their cytoplasmic PAD V deiminates histone H2A, H3, and H4 (other than nucleophosmin/B23). Cuthbert et al. (2004) and Wang et al. (2004) reported that PAD4 (correspondent to PAD V described by Yamada) deiminates histone H3 and H4 and has an impact on gene transcription by fine tuning the chromatin structure. In particular, Cuthbert et al. (2004) showed that PAD is activated when it is bound intracellularly by estrogen receptor. PAD deiminates histone H3 and H4 in different arginine located preferably in the N-terminal tail and increases the affinity of estrogen receptor for its target genes, thus resulting in a decrease of gene expression under the control of estrogen and thyroid hormones. When PAD4 activity is inhibited by Cl-amidine, an increase in the expression of p53- and p53 related genes is observed as described by Wang et al. (2004). PAD4 is not the only PAD isoform involved in chromatin regulation. Indeed, Zhang et al. (2012) suggested that stimulation of ERα-positive cells with 17β-estradiol (E2) promotes global citrullination of histone H3 arginine 26 (H3R26) on chromatin, catalyzed by PAD2 and not by PAD4, which instead deiminates H4R3. Importantly, deimination may involve arginine but also methylarginine on H4 and H3 induced by PRMT1 and CARM1, respectively, thus dubbing PAD4 as a demethylating enzyme, thereby reverting the epigenetic modification of arginine methylation. Like core histones, extranucleosomal linker histones can also be the target of PAD activity. Christophorou et al. (2014) recently demonstrated that H1 can also be citrullinated. Dwivedi et al. (2014) demonstrated that H1 is an additional substrate for PAD4, providing evidence that during NETosis a variety of linker H1 can be deiminated on multiple arginines. Notably, H1.2 is deiminated on arginine 53, and the neo-formed epitope is thus recognized by specific anticitrulline antibodies present in a small percentage of SLE and Sjögren's syndrome (SS) patients but not in RA For instance, the antibody-detecting citrulline after chemical modification with antipyrine and 2,3-butanedione, the so called "Senshuo reagent," also recognizes carbamylated proteins.

Citrullinated histones as autoantigens in rheumatoid arthritis

As discussed earlier core histones are the most abundant proteins in NET (Urban et al., 2009). Precisely deiminated histones are a target of antibodies in RA. Presence of antideiminated histone H3 antibodies has been detected

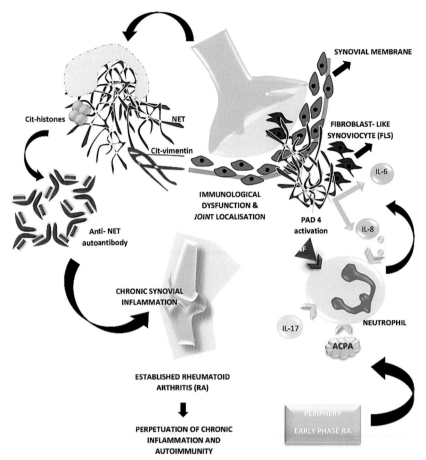

FIGURE 5.1   Role of NETosis in RA progression. Citrullination plays a prominent role in RA. Neutrophils can be activated by a vast number of stimulants (cytokines, TLR ligands, etc.) for NET formation. Neutrophils migrate across the periphery followed by excess NETosis leading to the generation of deiminated antigens, for example, citH2A, citH2B, and citH4 histones. These citrullinated antigens can be presented by APCs after ingestion of nuclear components of neutrophils. This continues presentation of citrullinated antigens and leads to antigen-driven autoimmune responses in the RA joint leading to anti-NET autoantibody generation which contributes to the prolongation of chronic inflammation and autoimmunity.

in sera from RA patients (Fig. 5.1). Autoantibodies specific for H4-derived citrullinated peptides HCP1—H414−34 and HCP2—H431−50 are present in 67% and 63% of established RA, respectively (Pratesi et al., 2014). The frequency is lower in early RA (37.3% and 48.5%, respectively), but they can be detected years before disease onset. Based on one of the major ACPA subtypes, anticitrullinated histone antibodies prime symptoms of RA and help to predict disease development (Johansson et al., 2016). Interestingly, antibodies against citrullinated sequences of H2A and H2B have been detected in healthy subjects that later develop RA. An enhancement in antibody frequency, together with the production of inflammatory cytokines, predicts the progression of clinically active RA (Sokolove et al., 2012). Furthermore, citrullinated H2B has been detected as a target of autoantibodies in a high number of patients with RA (Sohn et al., 2015). It has been observed that RA synovial fluids contain high levels of citH2B and its immune complex, which have proinflammatory and immunostimulatory capacity. Reports also suggest that immunization with citrullinated antigens like collagen II can boost tissue injury and stimulate ACPA production in experimental arthritis (Kuhn et al., 2006; Uysal et al., 2009), and that administration of anticitrullinated fibrinogen in collagen-induced arthritis enhances tissue injury (Kuhn et al., 2006).

Ectopic lymphoid structures as a source of antineutrophil extracellular trap antibodies in rheumatoid arthritis

Ectopic lymphoid structures (ELS) are formed due to infiltration of cluster of lymphomononuclear cells in the synovium fluids of RA joints. Synovial ELS are able to support a germinal center (GC) response. ELS are characterized by disintegration of T and B lymphocytes, differentiation of high endothelial venules, and complex of stromal follicular dendritic cells (Corsiero, Pitzalis, & Bombardieri, 2014; Manzo, Bombardieri, Humby, & Pitzalis, 2010). In RA patients, this ectopic GC induces the production of antibodies against citrullinated proteins (Croia et al., 2013; Humby et al., 2009; Masson-Bessiere et al., 2000), unlike other autoimmune diseases, whereas autoantibodies are generated against other antigens, that is, in myasthenia gravis antibodies are generated against acetylcholine receptor (Berrih-Aknin, Ragheb, Le Panse, & Lisak, 2013), in SS antibodies are generated against ribonucleoprotein Ro/La (Croia et al., 2014; Salomonsson et al., 2003), and in Hashimoto's thyroiditis antibodies are generated against thyroglobulin and thyroperoxidase (Armengol et al., 2001). Cell-based NET localization assay validates the presence of autoantibodies against histones in either synovial fluid or circulating neutrophils in RA patients. Therefore these antibodies are referred as anti-NET antibodies. Affinity maturation in these anti-NET antibodies takes place in the ectopic GC and is enriched by synovial microenvironment (Corsiero, Bombardieri, et al., 2016; Corsiero, Pratesi, Prediletto, Bombardieri, and Migliorini, 2016).

Environmental factors such as bacterial infection and smoking also lead to generation of ACPA in RA. Periodontal disease (i.e., *P. gingivalis*) (Lee et al., 2015; Wegner et al., 2010) and smoking (Kokkonen et al., 2015) can bring to the formation of citrullinated antigens outside the joints and can lead to ACPA production before the clinical preceding of the disease. Of interest, *P. gingivalis* is the only reported pathogen which expresses PAD, to citrullinate both the endogenous and host proteins, helping in ACPA formation (Li et al., 2016; White, Chicca, Cooper, Milward, & Chapple, 2015).

Bronchial biopsies from early RA patients provide evidence in support of the presence of inflammatory infiltrate containing T cells, B cells, and plasma cells and GC-like structures (Reynisdottir et al., 2016). Enhanced content of citrullinated proteins in synovial fluid, periodontal tissue, and the lung strongly suggests the occurrence of NETosis in RA patients, and the presence of ectopic GCs. It is well proved that increased concentration of NET-associated proteins due to upregulation of NET production or inefficient clearance of citrullinated autoantigens from circulation is able to trigger an autoimmune response. NETs reveal originated citrullinated proteins cathelicidin or high mobility group box 1 protein (HMGB1) together with danger signals that promote the activation and maturation of professional APCs. Activated APCs engulf NETs and further process it. This function of APCs facilitates the expansion of T cells and also supports the affinity maturation and clonal diversification of B cells.

Role of NETosis generated cell-free DNA in rheumatoid arthritis

Cell-free DNA (cfDNA) is an another major outcome of NETosis and also has deleterious effect in RA progression. It is an inducer of inflammation-triggering autoimmune responses. Accumulation of cfDNA and triggering immune response against it depend on inefficient clearance of NET components from circulation (Khandpur et al., 2013; Corsiero, Bombardieri, et al., 2016; Corsiero, Pratesi, et al., 2016). CfDNA is able to activate TLR-mediated immune responses and it also accelerates the production of antibodies against citrullinated antigens and antinuclear antigens. Antibodies further activate TLRs and B cells, and this activation cascade leads to the production of cytokines and chemokines. Microbial lipopeptides play an active role in the generation of TNF and IL-17 resulting into inflammation in RA patients. Recent studies reveal that there is increase in levels of cfDNA, cfRNA, and antibodies against them during RA condition (Zimmermann-Geller et al., 2016).

In conclusion it is well defined that NETosis plays an active role in pathogenesis of RA along with other autoimmune disease and serum concentrations of such NETosis-derived cytokines and autoantibodies in suspected RA cases might serve as a new complementary diagnostic tool.

Therapeutics based on modulating NETosis in rheumatoid arthritis

Triptolide (TP) proves to be potential effect as antiarthiritic mechanism. Recent studies in mice model of RA have shown the impact of TP in adjuvant-induced arthritis (AA) murine model of RA TP lightened AA by lowering neutrophil recruitment and it also downregulates the expression of interleukin-6 and tumor necrosis factor-α. TP is also able to suppress the expression of proinflammatory cytokines in neutrophils, also promotes neutrophil apoptosis and inhibits the migration, NETosis, and autophagy of neutrophils. Therefore TP represents a potential therapeutic agent for RA (Huang et al., 2018). Similarly, Tocilizumab also shows potential for reducing autoantibodies in serum level in RA patients (Ruiz-Limón et al., 2017).

NETosis in systemic lupus erythematosus

SLE is a multifactorial autoimmune disease affecting different organs, and is most prevalent in women of childbearing age. The molecular hallmarks of SLE are the formation of a distinct range of autoantibodies against nuclear and cytoplasmic elements and upregulation of type I interferon—regulated genes. It shows immense heterogeneity in both their autoantibody and clinical manifestations with the most abundant class of autoantibody generated being against double-stranded DNA (dsDNA). In SLE, NETs serve to aggravate the disease by triggering autoantibody against autoantigens like self-dsDNA, citrullinated histones, neutrophil elastase, etc. (Apel, Zychlinsky, & Kenny, 2018).

Neutrophil extracellular trap components in systemic lupus erythematosus

It has been reported that NET proteins are mainly ubiquitinated and autoantibodies against ubiquitinated MPO has been encountered in SLE patients. Normally monocyte-derived macrophages internalize prepossessed NET components. This prepossessing is performed by endonuclease DNase I. After being engulfed NETs are transported to lysosome via phagosome for degradation. Monocyte-derived macrophages are stimulated with ubiquitinated NET proteins to increase calcium influx in cells. This induces enhanced production of cytokines like TNF-α and IL-10, which further inhibits clearance of NET components by macrophages in SLE patients. This impaired clearance of NETs results in accumulation of self-dsDNA. In healthy individuals, macrophages actively participate in clearance of NET components without secreting proinflammatory cytokines and without harming the body. Inefficient NET clearance by macrophages results into excessive amount of NET proteins including dsDNA in SLE patients. However, the mechanisms by which NET proteins reach to the GC and trigger autoantibody production is not well understood (Barrera-Vargas et al., 2018).

Role of DNase I

DNase I, which is a major endonuclease in circulation, plays the prime role in NET-degradation (Hakkim et al., 2010). It has been found that SLE patients have low DNase I activity in their serum as compared to normal individuals (Fig. 5.2). DNase I—deficient mouse develops typical symptoms

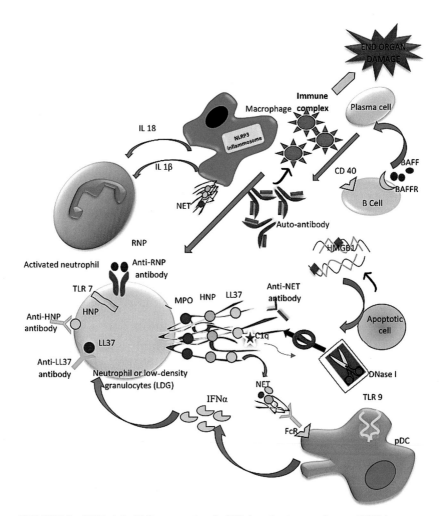

FIGURE 5.2   NETosis in SLE progression. In SLE, low-density granulocytes (LDGs) generate spontaneous NETs, when they are induced by anti-HNP or LL37 autoantibodies or RNP/anti-RNP immune complexes followed by TLR7 induction. Presence of DNase I inhibitory factors in the SLE serum (such as NET-associated anti-NET Abs, LL37, or C1q) inhibits degradation of NETs. Stimulation of pDC through FcRIIa and TLR9 leads to NET engulfment leading to secretion of IFNα. Consecutively, IFNα primes neutrophils for excess NETosis by upregulating TLR7 along with surface granular proteins (such as LL37 and HNP). T- and B-cell activation by IFNα provokes production of anti-NET Abs, such as anti-dsDNA, anti-LL37, and anti-HNP Abs. NETs also activate the NLRP3 inflammasome in macrophages to trigger the synthesis of IL-1β and IL-18. These two, in turn, can induce NETosis. These crosstalks between molecular loops summarize into a disturbed immune homeostasis that leads to autoimmune response in SLE pathogenesis.

of SLE, such as the presence of antinuclear antibody specifically against dsDNA, the presence of immune complexes in glomeruli. It has been reported that missense mutations in DNase I (Bodaño, Amarelo, González, Gómez-Reino, & Conde, 2004) and DNase1L3 also known as DNase gamma (Al-Mayouf et al., 2011) causes familial case of SLE, whereas mutations in DNases lead to lupus—like disease in mice (Napirei et al., 2000; Sisirak et al., 2016). NETs contain oxidized DNA in the form of 8-hydroxyguanosine, which protects DNA from degradation by endonucleases. Therefore deposition of excess self-dsDNA is SLE patients indicates inefficient DNase activity (Gehrke et al., 2013). Anti-NET antibodies, complement component C1q, act as DNase I inhibitor, by protecting NET from degradation (Hakkim et al., 2010; Leffler et al., 2012). C1q deposits upon NETs to protect them from degradation. Antimicrobial peptides LL37, or HMGB1, binding to NETs also interferes with NETs degradation mediated by DNase I. Presence of globular actin (G-actin) and anti-DNase I antibodies is also detected in sera of SLE patients (Leffler et al., 2012; Yeh, Chang, Liang, Wu, & Liu, 2003). So it can be concluded that impaired DNase I activity leads to accumulation of autoantigens of NET triggering SLE pathogenesis.

Neutrophil extracellular traps drive plasmacytoid dendritic cells to produce type I interferon in systemic lupus erythematosus

Type I interferons play a major role in SLE pathogenesis (Fig. 5.2). High level of type I interferons is noticed in the sera of SLE patients and positively correlates with disease prognosis (Hooks et al., 1979; Ytterberg and Schnitzer, 1982). A large number of IFN-inducible genes are found to be upregulated in peripheral blood mononuclear cells of SLE patients (Baechler et al., 2003; Bennett et al., 2003). Type I interferons elicit differentiation of plasmacytoid dendritic cells (pDCs) from monocytes upon interacting with NET autoantigens. Thus it executes the breakdown of peripheral tolerance in SLE. These IFN-induced DCs proficiently present autoantigens to helper T cells, resulting in abnormal expansion of autoreactive T and B cells (Barrat et al., 2005). Lande et al. (2011) reported that immune complex containing DNA and antimicrobial peptides, such as LL37 and human neutrophil peptide (HNP), also activates pDCs with the production of IFNα.

Low-density granulocytes have heightened capacity to make neutrophil extracellular traps

Along with IFN signature, SLE patients also show a distinct neutrophil signature in their peripheral blood. This definite signature of granulopoiesis is due to the presence of low-density granulocytes (LDGs) in PBMCs. It has been reported that LDGs have impaired phagocytic functions. LDGs have an increased tendency to from NETs as compared to normal neutrophil (Fig. 5.2). There are evidences showing the high population of LDGs present in SLE patients. Villanueva et al. (2011) reported through gene array experiments that LDGs from SLE patients have high number of antibacterial proteins and alarmins as compared to normal density SLE and control neutrophils. In addition, enhanced NET formation by LDGs is also reported in SLE. Higher NET formation leads to increased exposure of NETs antigen including LL37, dsDNA along with proinflammatory cytokines resulting into impairment of endothelium ensuing into vascular damages. Therefore LDGs can serve as marker of SLE and their presence positively associates with skin lesions and vasculitis in SLE patients.

Neutrophil extracellular traps mediate enhanced inflammasome activation in systemic lupus erythematosus

Inflammasomes are multiprotein complexes that encounter pathogenic threats and lead to activation and release of proinflammatory cytokines IL-1β and IL-18 (Lamkanfi and Dixit, 2012) mediated by the activation of caspase-1 (Fig. 5.2). NET and NET-associated autoantigens are able to activate the inflammasome system (Kahlenberg, Carmona-Rivera, Smith, & Kaplan, 2013). It has been reported that LPS-primed primary macrophages get activated when interacting with NET or LL37, which lead to the activation of the central enzyme Caspase-1 in inflammasomes resulting into secretion IL-1β and IL-18 (Kahlenberg et al., 2013). LL37 promotes the aggregation of Nod-like receptor family, pyrin domain-containing three protein (NLRP3) in inflammasome of macrophages (Kahlenberg et al., 2013). In addition, NET and LL37-induced inflammasome activation is increased in SLE patients than control which also leads to increased IL-18 secretion (Calvani, Richards, Tucci, Pannarale, & Silvestris, 2004; Kahlenberg et al., 2011). Consecutively, both the secreted IL-1β and IL-18 also induce NET formation, forming a feedback loop which facilitates the disease pathogenesis in SLE (Kahlenberg et al., 2013; Mitroulis et al., 2011).

Impaired neutrophil extracellular trap degradation in systemic lupus erythematosus

It is known that SLE patients cannot clear NETs, leading to the pathogenesis of lupus nephritis. Hakkim et al. (2010) have shown in their studies that serum endonuclease DNase1 is essential for NETs degradation. They observed that there was inefficient degradation of NETs by sera of a specific SLE subset. This may allow persistence and exposure of NET components for long enough for the immune system to see them as autoantigens. Two mechanisms thought to be responsible for this impaired NET disassembly were proposed to be either the presence of DNase1 inhibitors or anti-NET antibodies blocking the access of DNase1 to NETs. Impairment of DNase1 function and poor NETs degradation correlated with kidney involvement suggesting it to be a useful indicator of renal involvement. However, the extent to which these clearance processes (NET-degradation) are operative in serologically distinguished subsets of SLE patients was established by Chauhan, Rai, Singh, Rai, and Rai (2015). In their report, they evaluated NET-degradation and neutrophil phagocytosis efficiency among SLE patients with different autoantibody specificities. SLE patients were classified into three subsets based on their autoantibody profile (anti-dsDNA, anti-ENA, or both) as determined by ELISA. NET-degradation and neutrophil-mediated phagocytosis by SLE and control sera were assessed. Significant differences in NET-degradation and phagocytosis in SLE patients with autoantibodies against dsDNA and ENA were observed. NET-degradation efficiency was significantly impaired in SLE patients with anti-dsDNA autoantibodies and not in those with anti-ENA autoantibodies. However, in contrast to NET-degradation, neutrophil-mediated phagocytosis was impaired in all three subsets independent of autoantibody specificity. These observations suggest that varying NET clearance mechanisms is operative in SLE subsets with anti-dsDNA or anti-ENA autoantibodies. Based on these observations it was proposed that therapies targeted at improving NET clearance could be effective in anti-dsDNA$^+$ SLE patients.

Neutrophil extracellular trap has protective role in drug-induced systemic lupus erythematosus

Kienhöfer et al. (2017) suggested that NETs can also mediate a protective role against drug-induced lupus. They investigated the role of neutrophils and NETs on a mouse model of lupus triggered by intraperitoneal injection of alkane pristane. Pristane-induced lupus was aggravated as seen from elevated levels of antinuclear autoantibodies (ANAs) and exacerbated glomerulonephritis, in two mouse strains which were genetically impaired for induction of NET formation, that is, NOX2-deficient (Ncf1-mutated) and PAD4-deficient mice. They observed reduction in ability to form pristane-induced NETs in vivo in both Ncf1-mutated and PAD4-deficient mice, although there were high levels of inflammatory mediators in the peritoneum. These findings corroborated with results of the study using a neutropenic mice model, which exhibited higher levels of ANAs, indicating that NETs and neutrophils have a regulatory function in lupus.

Role of mitochondrial DNA in neutrophil extracellular trap in systemic lupus erythematosus

Deposition of mitochondrial DNA (mtDNA) in NETs in renal biopsy specimen of lupus nephritis has been reported. Presence of high levels of mtDNA in NETs, and anti-mtDNA antibody levels, was detected in SLE patients compared with controls and it correlated significantly with IFN scores and the disease activity index. Interestingly, mtDNA has great potential to trigger IFNα production from pDCs via TLRs. Metformin has shown positive effect in downregulation of the NET mtDNA−PDC−IFNα pathway. Metformin causes diminution of PMA-induced NET formation and CpG-stimulated PDC IFNα generation. Therefore metformin has the capacity to cure SLE patients by depressing NET efficacy (Wang, Li, Chen, Gu, & Ye, 2015).

Neutrophil extracellular trap−based therapeutics in neutrophil extracellular traps

Effect of inhibition of JAK on NETosis and systemic lupus erythematosus

Tofacitinib has been shown to play a beneficial role in SLE by targeting JAK1 and JAK3 in mice models of lupus. Tofacitinib mainly affects adaptive immune cells specifically by reducing CD8 + and double negative (DN) T cells. It has been reported that high numbers of CD8 + T cells are associated with disease activity and may lead to autoantigen generation through perforin/granzyme-related pathways in SLE (Blanco et al., 2005). Type I IFNs production by endogenous nucleic acids is an early event that primes immune dysregulation and develops autoimmunity. Therefore drugs that target the type I IFN pathway are mostly being investigated (Kirou and Gkrouzman, 2013). Type I IFNs signal through the JAK/STAT pathway. Therefore inhibition of this pathway by tofacitinib can lead to pleiotropic effects regulating dysregulation of innate and adaptive immune responses including priming of neutrophils to undergo NET formation, alterations in B-cell ontogeny, and improvement in lupus vasculopathy. Tofacitinib regulates NET formation and increases endothelium-dependent vasorelaxation and endothelial differentiation drastically. Therefore this drug is effective for both preventive and therapeutic strategies.

Effect of B cells−inhibiting drugs in NETosis

Immune complexes are also capable of triggering NET formation in vitro in SLE. Rituximab (RTX; anti-CD20) and Belimumab (BLM, anti-BAFF) are used in the treatment of autoimmune diseases including SLE, their effect has been investigated in NET formation. It has been reported that RTX and BLM effectively reduce ANAs and also regressed excessive NET formation ex vivo. It has been suggested that B-cell targeting by RTX and BLM indirectly regulates NET formation by neutrophils. RTX and BLM treatment showed preferential reductions of autoantibody levels compared to physiological antibody levels suggesting that autoantibody-secreting plasma cells are more susceptible to RTX and BLM (Kraaij et al., 2018).

Neutrophil extracellular traps in multiple sclerosis

MS is an autoimmune, chronic inflammatory, demyelinating disease of the central nervous system involving secondary neurodegeneration. It is the most common cause of neurological disability among young adults affecting more than 2 million people worldwide. The etiology of MS involves both complex genetic trait and environmental factors (Sospedra and Martin, 2005). Th17 cells (Tzartos et al., 2008) and autoreactive CD4$^+$ Th1 (Olsson et al., 1990) cells are considered to have a central role in disease progression. Th17 cells are involved in neutrophil-mediated proinflammatory responses (Pelletier et al., 2010), and neutrophil priming (Ziaber et al., 1998), neutrophils expressing higher levels of medullasin (Aoki, Miyatake, Shimizu, & Yoshida, 1984), or elevated neutrophil neutral protease has been described (Guarnieri, Lolli, & Amaducci, 1985) in MS patients during clinical relapses. Interestingly, studies in the mouse model for MS, experimental autoimmune, suggest that neutrophils play an important pathogenic role in encephalomyelitis (Carlson, Kroenke, Rao, Lane, & Segal, 2008; McColl et al., 1998).

Higher circulating levels of neutrophil extracellular traps in sera from relapsing-remitting multiple sclerosis patients

NETosis is also involved in pathogenesis of MS as it has been observed that neutrophils in MS and relapsing-remitting multiple sclerosis (RRMS) patients have higher tendency to undergo degranulation, oxidative burst, and release of NET as compared to healthy controls. The elevated amount of NETs leads to accumulation of autoantigens and resulting into inflammation (Fig. 5.3). The proportion of NET proteins (neutrophils elastase, CD63) is also found to be present in higher amount in MS patients or patients with MS in relapse due to neutrophil degranulation. NET formation in MS can be triggered by inflammatory mediators, such as IL-8, and, although NETs are the most efficient in eliminating pathogens, abnormally high production of NETs can be associated with pathophysiological conditions. Although NETosis is a defense mechanism of neutrophils playing a protective role for the host, but in MS it is associated with autoimmune response by provoking autoantibodies. PAD4 overexpression leads to abrupt generation of citrullinated proteins. Autoantibodies against these citrullinated autoantigens trigger the autoimmune response. It is well documented that delayed apoptosis leads to accumulation of NET components in MS patients leading to induction of autoimmunity (Naegele et al., 2012). The high amount of cathepsin G, elastase, causes increased T-cell activation and tissue damage contributing into MS pathogenesis (Tani, Murphy, Chertov, Oppenheim, & Wang, 2001). An another study by Myronovkij et al. (2016) identified an unconventional myosin IC (Myo1C) which is ubiquitously present in vertebrates and was found to be present in elevated levels in MS patients. The possible reason for

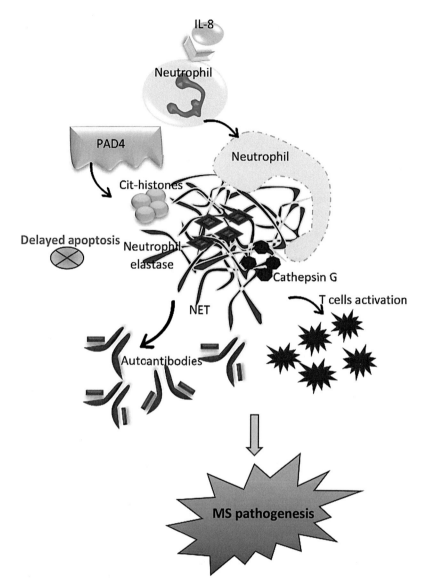

FIGURE 5.3   Effect of NETs in MS pathogenesis. In MS patients, neutrophils are in hyperactive conditions as they undergo degranulation, oxidative burst, and NET formation. Due to delay in apoptosis, released NETs components persist in the circulation resulting into the accumulation of autoantibodies against citrullinated proteins. Antimicrobial proteins (NE, Cathepsin G) secreted from NETosis causes increased T-cell activation leading to tissue damage in MS pathogenesis.

Myo1C abundance could be excessive NET formation in MS patients. Therefore proteolytic fragment of Myo1C could serve as a quantitative marker of NETosis in autoimmune conditions as Myo1C is also present in SLE and RA patients.

Neutrophil extracellular trap exhibits gender-specific difference in pathogenesis of multiple sclerosis

An interesting feature of NETs in MS condition is that NETs have gender-specific effects in pathogenesis as high levels of circulating NETs are observed in males with RRMS. As frequency of males affected by this disease is generally higher than that of females, the results suggest that NETosis may be at the core of some of the gender-specific differences in this disease and be involved in some aspects of MS pathogenesis such as breaching of the blood−brain barrier (Tillack et al., 2013).

Significantly higher levels of NETs are found in the serum of MS patients and it is speculated that these may be involved in MS pathogenesis. A large cohort of MS patients including patients suffering from other forms of MS other than RRMS were analyzed, and it was observed that only a small subset of RRMS patients has increased amount of circulating NETs. In addition, women of reproductive age have higher systemic neutrophil levels as compared with men, it is a relevant observation as RRMS mostly affects women around twice as much as men, but it has been found that male RRMS patients have high NETs in serum. However, no gender-specific differences have been reported in neutrophil counts and primed state. This highlights the role of gender-specific differences in pathogenesis of MS in RRMS patients although higher circulating NET levels do not seem to be a general feature of RRMS patients. MS is a highly complex disease involving very diverse pathomechanisms. Neutrophils are normally not present in the CNS of MS patients, this phenomenon of higher circulating NETs in some RRMS patients specifically in males could reflect a modification in NET formation or in NET-degradation. Although no differences in NETosis were observed between purified neutrophils from RRMS and healthy control and neither gender-specific significant differences. However, male RRMS patients exhibit significantly higher cell-free dsDNA in serum as compared to female patients suggesting an abnormal DNAse activity. This can be attributed to the higher circulating NET levels in male RRMS patients. However, in SLE, in which women are 10 times more frequently affected than men, it is found that the males are associated with more severe diseases and also with higher prevalence of pathogenic anti-dsDNA autoantibodies (Freire de Carvalho, do Nascimento, Testagrossa, Toledo-Barros, & Bonfa, 2010; Lu, Wallace, Ishimori, Scofield, & Weisman, 2010; Molina et al., 1996). Similarly, women are affected by RRMS about twice as often as men, and overall male gender has also been associated with worse prognosis.

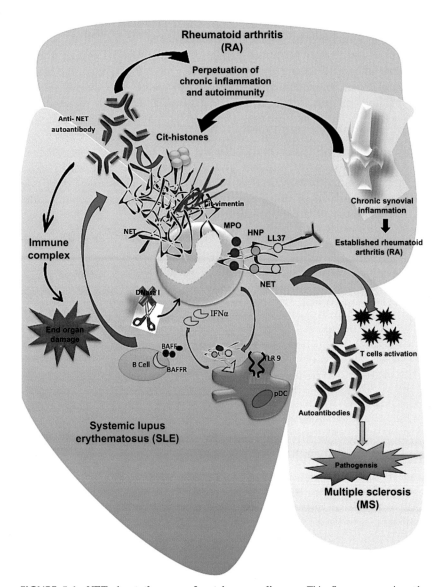

FIGURE 5.4   NETosis at the core of autoimmune diseases. This figure summarizes the involvement of NETs in RA, SLE, and MS. Citrullinated histones are the most abundant NET proteins targeted by autoantibodies, here, neutrophils cross the periphery to affect joints resulting into autoimmune conditions. In SLE, low-density granulocytes (LDGs) perform excessive NETosis leading to the generation of elevated amount of autoantibodies produced by B cells. These autoantibodies bind with specific antigens (NET proteins) to form immune complexes which accumulate in the kidney resulting in kidney damage. Next, immune complexes also activated pDCs by TLR induction to produce type I interferons which cause more NET formation. In MS patients, autoantibodies against NET components have detrimental effect in MS progression, higher T-cell activation by antimicrobial proteins generated from NETs also causes tissue destructions.

Interestingly, some reports have suggested that men with MS are prone to develop less inflammatory but more detrimental lesions than women (Pozzilli et al., 2003). The higher amount of circulating NET primes T cells and other immune cells and also regulates their migration through the blood−brain barrier and, consequently leads to more detrimental neuro-inflammatory processes in male RRMS patients. It has been reported that levels of NETs fluctuate over time in serum. This might be associated with disease activity but no correlation could be drawn between relapses and higher circulating NETs in serum (Tillack et al., 2013).

To conclude, it can be said that NETosis has an important role to play in the progression and pathogenesis of various autoimmune diseases (Fig. 5.4) and the development of drugs targeted at NET components could be the future of autoimmune disease management.

References

Al-Mayouf, S., Sunker, A., Abdwani, R., Abrawi, S., Almurshedi, F., Alhashmi, N., ... Alkuraya, F. (2011). Loss-of-function variant in DNASE1L3 causes a familial form of systemic lupus erythematosus. *Nature Genetics, 43*(12), 1186−1188.

Amara, K., Steen, J., Murray, F., Morbach, H., Fernandez-Rodriguez, B., Joshua, V., ... Malmström, V. (2013). Monoclonal IgG antibodies generated from joint-derived B cells of RA patients have a strong bias toward citrullinated autoantigen recognition. *The Journal of Experimental Medicine, 210*(3), 445−455.

Aoki, Y., Miyatake, T., Shimizu, N., & Yoshida, M. (1984). Medullasin activity in granulocytes of patients with multiple sclerosis. *Annals of Neurology, 15*(3), 245−249.

Apel, F., Zychlinsky, A., & Kenny, E. (2018). The role of neutrophil extracellular traps in rheumatic diseases. *Nature Reviews Rheumatology, 14*(8), 467−475.

Armengol, M., Juan, M., Lucas-Martín, A., Fernández-Figueras, M., Jaraquemada, D., Gallart, T., & Pujol-Borrell, R. (2001). Thyroid autoimmune disease. *The American Journal of Pathology, 159*(3), 861−873.

Asaga, H., Yamada, M., & Senshu, T. (1998). Selective deimination of vimentin in calcium ionophore-induced apoptosis of mouse peritoneal macrophages. *Biochemical and Biophysical Research Communications, 243*(3), 641−646.

Baechler, E., Batliwalla, F., Karypis, G., Gaffney, P., Ortmann, W., Espe, K., ... Behrens, T. (2003). Interferon-inducible gene expression signature in peripheral blood cells of patients with severe lupus. *Proceedings of the National Academy of Sciences, 100*(5), 2610−2615.

Barrat, F., Meeker, T., Gregorio, J., Chan, J., Uematsu, S., Akira, S., ... Coffman, R. (2005). Nucleic acids of mammalian origin can act as endogenous ligands for Toll-like receptors and may promote systemic lupus erythematosus. *The Journal of Experimental Medicine, 202* (8), 1131−1139.

Barrera-Vargas, A., Gómez-Martín, D., Carmona-Rivera, C., Merayo-Chalico, J., Torres-Ruiz, J., Manna, Z., ... Kaplan, M. (2018). Differential ubiquitination in NETs regulates macrophage responses in systemic lupus erythematosus. *Annals of the Rheumatic Diseases, 77*(6), 944−950.

Begovich, A., Carlton, V., Honigberg, L., Schrodi, S., Chokkalingam, A., Alexander, H., ... Gregersen, P. (2004). A missense single-nucleotide polymorphism in a gene encoding a protein tyrosine phosphatase (PTPN22) is associated with rheumatoid arthritis. *The American Journal of Human Genetics*, *75*(2), 330−337.

Bennett, L., Palucka, A., Arce, E., Cantrell, V., Borvak, J., Banchereau, J., & Pascual, V. (2003). Interferon and granulopoiesis signatures in systemic lupus erythematosus blood. *The Journal of Experimental Medicine*, *197*(6), 711−723.

Berrih-Aknin, S., Ragheb, S., Le Panse, R., & Lisak, R. (2013). Ectopic germinal centers, BAFF and anti-B-cell therapy in myasthenia gravis. *Autoimmunity Reviews*, *12*(9), 885−893.

Bizzaro, N., Bartoloni, E., Morozzi, G., Manganelli, S., Riccieri, V., Sabatini, P., ... Gerli, R. (2013). Anti-cyclic citrullinated peptide antibody titer predicts time to rheumatoid arthritis onset in patients with undifferentiated arthritis: Results from a 2-year prospective study. *Arthritis Research and Therapy*, *15*(1), R16.

Blanco, P., Pitard, V., Viallard, J. F., Taupin, J. L., Pellegrin, J. L., & Moreau, J. F. (2005). Increase in activated CD8 + T lymphocytes expressing perforin and granzyme B correlates with disease activity in patients with systemic lupus erythematosus. *Arthritis and Rheumatism*, *52*(1), 201−211.

Bodaño, A., Amarelo, J., González, A., Gómez- Reino, J. J., & Conde, C. (2004). Novel DNASE I mutations related to systemic lupus erythematosus. *Arthritis and Rheumatology*, *50*(12), 4070−4071.

Brink, M., Hansson, M., Mathsson, L., Jakobsson, P., Holmdahl, R., Hallmans, G., ... Rantapää-Dahlqvist, S. (2013). Multiplex analyses of antibodies against citrullinated peptides in individuals prior to development of rheumatoid arthritis. *Arthritis & Rheumatism*, *65*(4), 899−910.

Calvani, N., Richards, H., Tucci, M., Pannarale, G., & Silvestris, F. (2004). Up-regulation of IL-18 and predominance of a Th1 immune response is a hallmark of lupus nephritis. *Clinical and Experimental Immunology*, *138*(1), 171−178.

Carlson, T., Kroenke, M., Rao, P., Lane, T. E., & Segal, B. (2008). The Th17-ELR + CXC chemokine pathway is essential for the development of central nervous system autoimmune disease. *The Journal of Experimental Medicine*, *205*(4), 811−823.

Caudrillier, A., Kessenbrock, K., Gilliss, B., Nguyen, J., Marques, M., Monestier, M., ... Looney, M. (2012). Platelets induce neutrophil extracellular traps in transfusion-related acute lung injury. *Journal of Clinical Investigation*, *122*(7), 2661−2671.

Chang, H., Dwivedi, N., Nicholas, A., & Ho, I. (2015). The W620 polymorphism in PTPN22 disrupts its interaction with peptidylarginine deiminase type 4 and enhances citrullination and NETosis. *Arthritis and Rheumatology*, *67*(9), 2323−2334.

Chauhan, S. K., Rai, R., Singh, V. V., Rai, M., & Rai, G. (2015). Differential clearance mechanisms, neutrophil extracellular trap degradation and phagocytosis, are operative in systemic lupus erythematosus patients with distinct autoantibody specificities. *Immunology Letters*, *168*(2), 254−259.

Christophorou, M., Castelo-Branco, G., Halley-Stott, R., Oliveira, C., Loos, R., Radzisheuskaya, A., ... Kouzarides, T. (2014). Citrullination regulates pluripotency and histone H1 binding to chromatin. *Nature*, *507*(7490), 104−108.

Corsiero, E., Bombardieri, M., Carlotti, E., Pratesi, F., Robinson, W., Migliorini, P., & Pitzalis, C. (2016). Single cell cloning and recombinant monoclonal antibodies generation from RA synovial B cells reveal frequent targeting of citrullinated histones of NETs. *Annals of the Rheumatic Disease*, *75*(10), 1866−1875. Available from https://doi.org/10.1136/annrheumdis-208356.

Corsiero, E., Pitzalis, C., & Bombardieri, M. (2014). Peripheral and synovial mechanisms of humoral autoimmunity in rheumatoid arthritis. *Drug Discovery Today*, *19*(8), 1161−1165.

Corsiero, E., Pratesi, F., Prediletto, E., Bombardieri, M., & Migliorini, P. (2016). NETosis as source of autoantigens in rheumatoid arthritis. *Frontiers in Immunology*, 7, 485. Available from https://doi.org/10.3389/fimmu.2016.00485.

Croia, C., Astorri, E., Murray-Brown, W., Willis, A., Brokstad, K., Sutcliffe, N., ... Bombardieri, M. (2014). Implication of Epstein-Barr virus infection in disease-specific autoreactive B cell activation in ectopic lymphoid structures of Sjögren's syndrome. *Arthritis and Rheumatology*, 66(9), 2545−2557.

Croia, C., Serafini, B., Bombardieri, M., Kelly, S., Humby, F., Severa, M., ... Pitzalis, C. (2013). Epstein−Barr virus persistence and infection of autoreactive plasma cells in synovial lymphoid structures in rheumatoid arthritis. *Annals of the Rheumatic Diseases*, 72(9), 1559−1568.

Cuthbert, G., Daujat, S., Snowden, A., Erdjument-Bromage, H., Hagiwara, T., Yamada, M., ... Kouzarides, T. (2004). Histone deimination antagonizes arginine methylation. *Cell*, 118(5), 545−553.

Darrah, E., Giles, J., Ols, M., Bull, H., Andrade, F., & Rosen, A. (2013). Erosive rheumatoid arthritis is associated with antibodies that activate PAD4 by increasing calcium sensitivity. *Science Translational Medicine*, 5(186). Available from https://doi.org/10.1126/scitranslmed.3005370, 186ra65.

Dwivedi, N., Neeli, I., Schall, N., Wan, H., Desiderio, D., Csernok, E., ... Radic, M. (2014). Deimination of linker histones links neutrophil extracellular trap release with autoantibodies in systemic autoimmunity. *The FASEB Journal*, 28(7), 2840−2851.

Freire de Carvalho, J., do Nascimento, A. P., Testagrossa, L. A., Toledo-Barros, R., & Bonfa, E. (2010). Male gender results in more severe lupus nephritis. *Rheumatology International*, 30, 1311−1315.

Froy, O., & Sthoeger, Z. M. (2009). Defensins in systemic lupus erythematosus. *Annals of the New York Academy of Science*, 1173, 365−369.

Gehrke, N., Mertens, C., Zillinger, T., Wenzel, J., Bald, T., Zahn, S., ... Barchet, W. (2013). Oxidative damage of DNA confers resistance to cytosolic nuclease TREX1 degradation and potentiates STING-dependent immune sensing. *Immunity*, 39(3), 482−495.

Giles, J., Fert-Bober, J., Park, J., Bingham, C., Andrade, F., Fox-Talbot, K., ... Halushka, M. (2012). Myocardial citrullination in rheumatoid arthritis: A correlative histopathologic study. *Arthritis Research and Therapy*, 14(1), R39.

Glant, T. T., Ocsko, T., Markovics, A., Szekanecz, Z., Katz, R. S., Rauch, T. A., & Mikecz, K. (2016). Characterization and localization of citrullinated proteoglycan aggrecan in human articular cartilage. *PLoS One*, 11(3), e0150784. Available from https://doi.org/10.1371/journal.pone.0150784.

Guarnieri, B., Lolli, F., & Amaducci, L. (1985). Polymorphonuclear neutral protease activity in multiple sclerosis and other diseases. *Annals of Neurology*, 18(5), 620−622.

Hagiwara, T., Hidaka, Y., & Yamada, M. (2005). Deimination of histone H2A and H4 at arginine 3 in HL-60 granulocytes. *Biochemistry*, 44(15), 5827−5834.

Hakkim, A., Furnrohr, B., Amann, K., Laube, B., Abed, U., Brinkmann, V., ... Zychlinsky, A. (2010). Impairment of neutrophil extracellular trap degradation is associated with lupus nephritis. *Proceedings of the National Academy of Sciences*, 107(21), 9813−9818.

Hooks, J., Moutsopoulos, H., Geis, S., Stahl, N., Decker, J., & Notkins, A. (1979). Immune interferon in the circulation of patients with autoimmune disease. *New England Journal of Medicine*, 301(1), 5−8.

Huang, G., Yuan, K., Zhu, Q., Zhang, S., Lu, Q., Zhu, M., ... Xu, A. (2018). Triptolide inhibits the inflammatory activities of neutrophils to ameliorate chronic arthritis. *Molecular Immunology*, 101, 210−220.

Humby, F., Bombardieri, M., Manzo, A., Kelly, S., Blades, M., Kirkham, B., . . . Pitzalis, C. (2009). Ectopic lymphoid structures support ongoing production of class-switched autoantibodies in rheumatoid synovium. *PLoS Medicine*, *6*(1), e1. Available from https://doi.org/10.1371/journal.pmed.0060001.

Iobagiu, C., Magyar, A., Nogueira, L., Cornillet, M., Sebbag, M., Arnaud, J., . . . Serre, G. (2011). The antigen specificity of the rheumatoid arthritis-associated ACPA directed to citrullinated fibrin is very closely restricted. *Journal of Autoimmunity*, *37*(4), 263−272.

Johansson, L., Pratesi, F., Brink, M., Ärlestig, L., D'Amato, C., Bartaloni, D., . . . Rantapää-Dahlqvist, S. (2016). Antibodies directed against endogenous and exogenous citrullinated antigens pre-date the onset of rheumatoid arthritis. *Arthritis Research and Therapy*, *18*(1), 127. Available from https://doi.org/10.1186/s13075-016-1031-0.

Jorch, S. K., & Kubes, P. (2017). An emerging role for neutrophil extracellular traps in noninfectious disease. *Nature Medicine*, *23*(3), 279−287. Available from https://doi.org/10.1038/nm.4294.

Kahlenberg, J., Carmona-Rivera, C., Smith, C., & Kaplan, M. (2013). Neutrophil extracellular trap-associated protein activation of the NLRP3 inflammasome is enhanced in lupus macrophages. *The Journal of Immunology*, *190*(3), 1217−1226.

Kahlenberg, J., Thacker, S., Berthier, C., Cohen, C., Kretzler, M., & Kaplan, M. (2011). Inflammasome activation of IL-18 results in endothelial progenitor cell dysfunction in systemic lupus erythematosus. *The Journal of Immunology*, *187*(11), 6143−6156.

Khandpur, R., Carmona-Rivera, C., Vivekanandan-Giri, A., Gizinski, A., Yalavarthi, S., Knight, J., . . . Kaplan, M. (2013). NETs are a source of citrullinated autoantigens and stimulate inflammatory responses in rheumatoid arthritis. *Science Translational Medicine*, *5*(178), 178ra40−178ra40.

Kienhöfer, D., Hahn, J., Stoof, J., Csepregi, J. Z., Reinwald, C., Urbonaviciute, V., . . . Hoffmann, M. H. (2017). Experimental lupus is aggravated in mouse strains with impaired induction of neutrophil extracellular traps. *Journal of Clinical Investigation Insight*, *2*(10), 1−13. Available from https://doi.org/10.1172/jci.insight.92920.

Kinloch, A., Lundberg, K., Wait, R., Wegner, N., Lim, N., Zendman, A., . . . Venables, P. (2008). Synovial fluid is a site of citrullination of autoantigens in inflammatory arthritis. *Arthritis & Rheumatism*, *58*(8), 2287−2295.

Kirou, K. A., & Gkrouzman, E. (2013). Anti-interferon alpha treatment in SLE. *Clinical Immunology*, *148*(3), 303−312.

Knight, J., Zhao, W., Luo, W., Subramanian, V., O'Dell, A., Yalavarthi, S., . . . Kaplan, M. (2013). Peptidylarginine deiminase inhibition is immunomodulatory and vasculoprotective in murine lupus. *Journal of Clinical Investigation*, *123*(7), 2981−2993.

Kokkonen, H., Brink, M., Hansson, M., Lassen, E., Mathsson-Alm, L., Holmdahl, R., . . . Rantapää-Dahlqvist, S. (2015). Associations of antibodies against citrullinated peptides with human leukocyte antigen-shared epitope and smoking prior to the development of rheumatoid arthritis. *Arthritis Research & Therapy*, *17*, 2−15.

Kraaij, T., Kamerling, S., de Rooij, E., van Daele, P., Bredewold, O., Bakker, J., . . . Teng, Y. (2018). The NET-effect of combining rituximab with belimumab in severe systemic lupus erythematosus. *Journal of Autoimmunity*, *91*, 45−54.

Kuhn, K. A., Kulik, L., Tomooka, B., Braschler, K. J., Arend, W. P., Robinson, W. H., & Holers, V. M. (2006). Antibodies against citrullinated proteins enhance tissue injury in experimental autoimmune arthritis. *Journal of Clinical Investigation*, *116*(4), 961−973. Available from https://doi.org/10.1172/JCI25422.

Lamkanfi, M., & Dixit, V. M. (2012). Inflammasomes and their roles in health and disease. *Annual Review of Cell and Developmental Biology*, *28*, 137−161.

Lande, R., Ganguly, D., Facchinetti, V., Frasca, L., Conrad, C., Gregorio, J., ... Gilliet, M. (2011). Neutrophils activate plasmacytoid dendritic cells by releasing self-DNA-peptide complexes in systemic lupus erythematosus. *Science Translational Medicine*, *3*(73), 73ra19−73ra19.

Lee, J., Choi, I., Kim, J., Kim, K., Lee, E., Lee, E., ... Song, Y. (2015). Association between anti-*Porphyromonas gingivalis* or anti-α enolase antibody and severity of periodontitis or rheumatoid arthritis (RA) disease activity in RA. *BMC Musculoskeletal Disorders*, *16*, 190. Available from https://doi.org/10.1186/s12891-015-0647-6.

Leffler, J., Martin, M., Gullstrand, B., Tyden, H., Lood, C., Truedsson, L., ... Blom, A. (2012). Neutrophil extracellular traps that are not degraded in systemic lupus erythematosus activate complement exacerbating the disease. *The Journal of Immunology*, *188*(7), 3522−3531.

Li, S., Yu, Y., Yue, Y., Liao, H., Xie, W., Thai, J., ... Su, K. (2016). Autoantibodies from single circulating plasmablasts react with citrullinated antigens and *Porphyromonas gingivalis* in rheumatoid arthritis. *Arthritis and Rheumatology*, *68*(3), 614−626.

Lu, L., Wallace, D., Ishimori, M., Scofield, R., & Weisman, M. (2010). Review: Male systemic lupus erythematosus: A review of sex disparities in this disease. *Lupus*, *19*(2), 119−129.

Lugli, E., Correia, R., Fischer, R., Lundberg, K., Bracke, K., Montgomery, A., ... Venables, P. (2015). Expression of citrulline and homocitrulline residues in the lungs of non-smokers and smokers: Implications for autoimmunity in rheumatoid arthritis. *Arthritis Research & Therapy*, *17*(1), 9. Available from https://doi.org/10.1186/s13075-015-0520-x.

Makrygiannakis, D., af Klint, E., Lundberg, I., Lofberg, R., Ulfgren, A., Klareskog, L., & Catrina, A. (2006). Citrullination is an inflammation-dependent process. *Annals of the Rheumatic Diseases*, *65*(9), 1219−1222.

Malmström, V., Catrina, A., & Klareskog, L. (2017). The immunopathogenesis of seropositive rheumatoid arthritis: From triggering to targeting. *Nature Reviews Immunology*, *17*(1), 60−75.

Manolova, I., Dancheva, M., & Halacheva, K. (2001). Antineutrophil cytoplasmic antibodies in patients with systemic lupus erythematosus: Prevalence, antigen specificity, and clinical associations. *Rheumatology International*, *20*(5), 197−204.

Mantovani, A., Cassatella, M., Costantini, C., & Jaillon, S. (2011). Neutrophils in the activation and regulation of innate and adaptive immunity. *Nature Reviews Immunology*, *11*(8), 519−531.

Manzo, A., Bombardieri, M., Humby, F., & Pitzalis, C. (2010). Secondary and ectopic lymphoid tissue responses in rheumatoid arthritis: From inflammation to autoimmunity and tissue damage/remodeling. *Immunological Reviews*, *233*(1), 267−285.

Masson-Bessiere, C., Sebbag, M., Durieux, J., Nogueira, L., Vincent, C., Girbal-Neuhauser, E., ... Serre, G. (2000). In the rheumatoid pannus, anti-filaggrin autoantibodies are produced by local plasma cells and constitute a higher proportion of IgG than in synovial fluid and serum. *Clinical and Experimental Immunology*, *119*(3), 544−552.

McColl, S. R., Staykova, M. A., Wozniak, A., Fordham, S., Bruce, J., & Willenborg, D. O. (1998). Treatment with anti-granulocyte antibodies inhibits the effector phase of experimental autoimmune encephalomyelitis. *Journal of Immunology*, *161*(11), 6421−6426.

Mitroulis, I., Kambas, K., Chrysanthopoulou, A., Skendros, P., Apostolidou, E., Kourtzelis, I., ... Ritis, K. (2011). Neutrophil extracellular trap formation is associated with IL-1β and autophagy-related signaling in gout. *PLoS One*, *6*, e29318.

Mohamed, B., Verma, N., Davies, A., McGowan, A., Crosbie-Staunton, K., Prina-Mello, A., ... Volkov, Y. (2012). Citrullination of proteins: A common post-translational modification pathway induced by different nanoparticlesin vitroandin vivo. *Nanomedicine*, *7*(8), 1181−1195.

Molina, J. F., Drenkard, C., Molina, J., Cardiel, M. H., Uribe, O., Anaya, J. M., ... Alarcon-Segovia, D. (1996). Systemic lupus erythematosus in males. A study of 107 Latin American patients. *Medicine (Baltimore)*, *75*(3), 124–130.

Myronovkij, S., Negrych, N., Nehrych, T., Redowicz, M., Souchelnytskyi, S., Stoika, R., & Kit, Y. (2016). Identification of a 48 kDa form of unconventional myosin 1c in blood serum of patients with autoimmune diseases. *Biochemistry and Biophysics Reports*, *5*, 175–179.

Naegele, M., Tillack, K., Reinhardt, S., Schippling, S., Martin, R., & Sospedra, M. (2012). Neutrophils in multiple sclerosis are characterized by a primed phenotype. *Journal of Neuroimmunology*, *242*(1–2), 60–71.

Napirei, M., Karsunky, H., Zevnik, B., Stephan, H., Mannherz, H., & Möröy, T. (2000). Features of systemic lupus erythematosus in Dnase1-deficient mice. *Nature Genetics*, *25*(2), 177–181.

Neeli, I., Khan, S., & Radic, M. (2008). Histone deimination as a response to inflammatory stimuli in neutrophils. *The Journal of Immunology*, *180*(3), 1895–1902.

Nishimura, K., Sugiyama, D., Kogata, Y., Tsuji, G., Nakazawa, T., Kawano, S., ... Kumagai, S. (2007). *Meta*-analysis: Diagnostic accuracy of anti–cyclic citrullinated peptide antibody and rheumatoid factor for rheumatoid arthritis. *Annals of Internal Medicine*, *146*(11), 797.

Olsson, T., Zhi, W. W., Hojeberg, B., Kostulas, V., Jiang, Y. P., Anderson, G., ... Link, H. (1990). Autoreactive T lymphocytes in multiple sclerosis determined by antigen- induced secretion of interferon-gamma. *Journal of Clinical Investigation*, *86*(3), 981–985.

Padyukov, L., Seielstad, M., Ong, R., Ding, B., Ronnelid, J., Seddighzadeh, M., ... Klareskog, L. (2011). A genome-wide association study suggests contrasting associations in ACPA-positive vs ACPA-negative rheumatoid arthritis. *Annals of the Rheumatic Diseases*, *70*(2), 259–265.

Pelletier, M., Maggi, L., Micheletti, A., Lazzeri, E., Tamassia, N., Costantini, C., ... Cassatella, M. A. (2010). Evidence for a cross-talk between human neutrophils and Th17 cells. *Blood*, *115*(2), 335–343.

Pozzilli, C., Tomassini, V., Marinelli, F., Paolillo, A., Gasperini, C., & Bastianello, S. (2003). 'Gender gap' inmultiple sclerosis: Magnetic resonance imaging evidence. *European Journal of Neurology*, *10*, 95–97.

Pradhan, V. D., Badakere, S. S., Bichile, L. S., & Almeida, A. F. (2004). Anti-neutrophil cytoplasmic antibodies (ANCA) in systemic lupus erythematosus: Prevalence, clinical associations and correlation with other autoantibodies. *The Journal of the Association of Physicians of India*, *2004*(52), 533–5377.

Pratesi, F., Dioni, I., Tommasi, C., Alcaro, M., Paolini, I., Barbetti, F., ... Migliorini, P. (2014). Antibodies from patients with rheumatoid arthritis target citrullinated histone 4 contained in neutrophils extracellular traps. *Annals of the Rheumatic Diseases*, *73*(7), 1414–1422.

Raychaudhuri, S., Sandor, C., Stahl, E., Freudenberg, J., Lee, H., Jia, X., ... de Bakker, P. (2012). Five amino acids in three HLA proteins explain most of the association between MHC and seropositive rheumatoid arthritis. *Nature Genetics*, *44*(3), 291–296.

Reynisdottir, G., Olsen, H., Joshua, V., Engström, M., Forsslund, H., Karimi, R., ... Catrina, A. (2016). Signs of immune activation and local inflammation are present in the bronchial tissue of patients with untreated early rheumatoid arthritis. *Annals of the Rheumatic Diseases*, *75*(9), 1722–1727.

Romero, V., Fert-Bober, J., Nigrovic, P., Darrah, E., Haque, U., Lee, D., ... Andrade, F. (2013). Immune-mediated pore-forming pathways induce cellular hypercitrullination and generate citrullinated autoantigens in rheumatoid arthritis. *Science Translational Medicine*, *5*(209). Available from https://doi.org/10.1126/scitranslmed.3006869, 209ra150.

Ruiz-Limón, P., Ortega, R., Arias de la Rosa, I., Abalos-Aguilera, M., Perez- Sanchez, C., Jimenez- Gomez, Y., ... Barbarroja, N. (2017). Tocilizumab improves the proatherothrombotic profile of rheumatoid arthritis patients modulating endothelial dysfunction, NETosis, and inflammation. *Translational Research*, *183*, 87−103.

Salomonsson, S., Jonsson, M. V., Skarstein, K., Brokstad, K. A., Hjelmstrom, P., Wahren-Herlenius, M., & Jonsson, R. (2003). Cellular basis of ectopic germinal center formation and autoantibody production in the target organ of patients with Sjogren's syndrome. *Arthritis and Rheumatism*, *48*(11), 3187−3201. Available from https://doi.org/10.1002/art.11311.

Schuerwegh, A., Ioan-Facsinay, A., Dorjee, A., Roos, J., Bajema, I., van der Voort, E., ... Toes, R. (2010). Evidence for a functional role of IgE anticitrullinated protein antibodies in rheumatoid arthritis. *Proceedings of the National Academy of Sciences*, *107*(6), 2586−2591.

Sisirak, V., Sally, B., D'Agati, V., Martinez-Ortiz, W., Özçakar, Z., David, J., ... Reizis, B. (2016). Digestion of chromatin in apoptotic cell microparticles prevents autoimmunity. *Cell*, *166*(1), 88−101.

Sohn, D., Rhodes, C., Onuma, K., Zhao, X., Sharpe, O., Gazitt, T., ... Sokolove, J. (2015). Local joint inflammation and histone citrullination in a murine model of the transition from preclinical autoimmunity to inflammatory arthritis. *Arthritis & Rheumatology*, *67*(11), 2877−2887.

Sokolove, J., Bromberg, R., Deane, K. D., Lahey, L. J., Derber, L. A., Chandra, P. E., ... Robinson, W. H. (2012). Autoantibody epitope spreading in the pre-clinical phase predicts progression to rheumatoid arthritis. *PLoS One*, *7*, e35296. Available from https://doi.org/10.1371/journal.pone.0035296.

Sospedra, M., & Martin, R. (2005). Immunology of multiple sclerosis. *Annual Review of Immunology*, *23*, 683−747.

Spengler, J., Lugonja, B., Jimmy Ytterberg, A., Zubarev, R., Creese, A., Pearson, M., ... Scheel-Toellner, D. (2015). Release of active peptidyl arginine deiminases by neutrophils can explain production of extracellular citrullinated autoantigens in rheumatoid arthritis synovial fluid. *Arthritis & Rheumatology*, *67*(3), 135−3145.

Stolt, P., Yahya, A., Bengtsson, C., Källberg, H., Rönnelid, J., Lundberg, I., ... EIRA Study Group. (2010). Silica exposure among male current smokers is associated with a high risk of developing ACPA-positive rheumatoid arthritis. *Annals of the Rheumatic Diseases*, *69*(6), 1072−1076.

Tamiya, H., Tani, K., Miyata, J., Sato, K., Urata, T., Lkhagvaa, B., ... Sone, S. (2006). Defensins- and cathepsin G-ANCA in systemic lupus erythematosus. *Rheumatology International*, *27*(2), 147−152.

Tani, K., Murphy, W. J., Chertov, O., Oppenheim, J. J., & Wang, J. M. (2001). The neutrophil granule protein cathepsin G activates murine T lymphocytes and upregulates antigen-specific IG production in mice. *Biochemical and Biophysical Research Communication*, *282*(4), 971−976.

Thomas, G. M., Carbo, C., Curtis, B. R., Martinod, K., Mazo, I. B., Schatzberg, D., ... Wagner, D. D. (2012). Extracellular DNA traps are associated with the pathogenesis of TRALI in humans and mice. *Blood*, *119*(26), 6335−6343.

Tillack, K., Naegele, M., Haueis, C., Schippling, S., Wandinger, K., Martin, R., & Sospedra, M. (2013). Gender differences in circulating levels of neutrophil extracellular traps in serum of multiple sclerosis patients. *Journal of Neuroimmunology*, *261*(1−2), 108−119.

Too, C. L., Muhamad, N. A., Ilar, A., Padyukov, L., Alfredsson, L., Klareskog, L., ... Bengtsson, C. (2016). Occupational exposure to textile dust increases the risk of rheumatoid arthritis: Results from a Malaysian population-based case-control study. *Annals of the Rheumatic Diseases*, *75*(6), 997−1002.

Tzartos, J. S., Friese, M. A., Craner, M. J., Palace, J., Newcombe, J., Esiri, M. M., & Fugger, L. (2008). Interleukin-17 production in central nervous system-infiltrating T cells and glial cells is associated with active disease in multiple sclerosis. *The American Journal of Pathology*, *172*(1), 146−155.

Urban, C. F., Ermert, D., Schmid, M., Abu-Abed, U., Goosmann, C., Nacken, W., ... Zychlinsky, A. (2009). Neutrophil extracellular traps contain calprotectin, a cytosolic protein complex involved in host defense against Candida albicans. *PLoS Pathogens*, *5*(10), e1000639. Available from https://doi.org/10.1371/journal.ppat.1000639.

Uysal, H., Bockermann, R., Nandakumar, K., Sehnert, B., Bajtner, E., Engström, Å., ... Holmdahl, R. (2009). Structure and pathogenicity of antibodies specific for citrullinated collagen type II in experimental arthritis. *The Journal of Experimental Medicine*, *206*(2), 449−462.

Villanueva, E., Yalavarthi, S., Berthier, C., Hodgin, J., Khandpur, R., Lin, A. M., ... Kaplan, M. J. (2011). Netting neutrophils induce endothelial damage, infiltrate tissues, and expose immunostimulatory molecules in systemic lupus erythematosus. *The Journal of Immunology*, *187*(1), 538−552.

Wang, H., Li, T., Chen, S., Gu, Y., & Ye, S. (2015). Neutrophil extracellular trap mitochondrial DNA and its autoantibody in systemic lupus erythematosus and a proof-of-concept trial of metformin. *Arthritis & Rheumatology*, *67*(12), 3190−3200.

Wang, Y., Wysocka, J., Sayegh, J., Lee, Y. H., Perlin, J. R., Leonelli, L., ... Coonrod, S. A. (2004). Human PAD4 regulates histone arginine methylation levels via demethylimination. *Science*, *306*(5694), 279−283. Available from https://doi.org/10.1126/science.1101400.

Wegner, N., Wait, R., Sroka, A., Eick, S., Nguyen, K., Lundberg, K., ... Venables, P. (2010). Peptidylarginine deiminase from *Porphyromonas gingivalis* citrullinates human fibrinogen and α-enolase: Implications for autoimmunity in rheumatoid arthritis. *Arthritis & Rheumatism*, *62*(9), 2662−2672.

Wei, L., Wasilewski, E., Chakka, S., Bello, A., Moscarello, M., & Kotra, L. (2013). Novel inhibitors of protein arginine deiminase with potential activity in multiple sclerosis animal model. *Journal of Medicinal Chemistry*, *56*(4), 1715−1722.

White, P., Chicca, I., Cooper, P., Milward, M., & Chapple, I. (2015). Neutrophil extracellular traps in periodontitis. *Journal of Dental Research*, *95*(1), 26−34.

Willis, V., Gizinski, A., Banda, N., Causey, C., Knuckley, B., Cordova, K., ... Holers, V. (2011). N-α-Benzoyl-N5-(2-chloro-1-iminoethyl)-l-ornithine amide, a protein arginine deiminase inhibitor, reduces the severity of murine collagen-induced arthritis. *The Journal of Immunology*, *186*(7), 4396−4404.

Yeh, T., Chang, H., Liang, C., Wu, J., & Liu, M. (2003). Deoxyribonuclease-inhibitory antibodies in systemic lupus erythematosus. *Journal of Biomedical Science*, *10*(5), 544−551.

Ytterberg, S., & Schnitzer, T. (1982). Serum interferon levels in patients with systemic lupus erythematosus. *Arthritis & Rheumatism*, *25*(4), 401−406.

Yu, Y., & Su, K. (2013). Neutrophil extracellular traps and systemic lupus erythematosus. *Journal of Clinical & Cellular Immunology*, *4*, 139. Available from https://doi.org/10.4172/2155-9899.1000139.

Zhang, X., Bolt, M., Guertin, M. J., Chen, W., Zhang, S., Cherrington, B. D., ... Coonrod, S. A. (2012). Peptidylarginine deiminase 2-catalyzed histone H3 arginine 26 citrullination facilitates estrogen receptor alpha target gene activation. *Proceedings of the National Academy of*

Sciences of the United States, 109(33), 13331−13336. Available from https://doi.org/10.1073/pnas.1203280109.

Ziaber, J., Pasnik, J., Baj, Z., Pokoca, L., Chmielewski, H., & Tchorzewski, H. (1998). The immunoregulatory abilities of polymorphonuclear neutrophils in the course of multiple sclerosis. *Mediators of Inflammation, 7*(5), 335−338.

Zimmermann-Geller, B., Köppert, S., Fischer, S., Cabrera-Fuentes, H. A., Lefèvre, S., Rickert, M., . . . Neumann, E. (2016). Influence of extracellular RNAs, released by rheumatoid arthritis synovial fibroblasts, on their adhesive and invasive properties. *Journal of Immunology, 197*(7), 2589−2597.

Chapter 6

NETosis in other diseases and therapeutic approaches

Neutrophils as innate immune phagocytes have a central role in immune response. The prime function of neutrophils was believed to be pathogen phagocytosis killing via fusion of granules containing lytic proteases with phagosomes. Web-like chromatin structures called neutrophil extracellular traps (NETs) were first reported in 2004 as a novel biophylactic mechanism. The development of NET is a defense mechanism utilized by neutrophils to trap and proficiently constrain the damage inflicted by a wide range of microbial targets. In addition to providing defense against pathogens to block their systemic dissemination during infection, NET production is also known to be associated with disorders like sterile inflammation, atherosclerosis, and occurrence of autoimmune diseases such as systemic lupus erythematosus.

Recent studies suggest the role of NET in infectious diseases as well as in cardiovascular diseases, autoimmunity, metabolic disorders, and cancer. In this chapter, the role of NET in cystic fibrosis (CF), diabetes, cancer, Alzheimer's disease (AD), gout, pancreatitis as well as infectious diseases will be discussed, with an exploration of the future prospective and therapeutic opportunities.

NETosis in cystic fibrosis

CF is a lung disease associated with chronic inflammation of the airways caused due to bacterial colonization. It is the most common life-threatening inherited disease which primarily affects the respiratory system, gastrointestinal tract, and the hepatobiliary, reproductive and musculoskeletal systems. It is an autosomal genetic disorder resulting from the mutation of cystic fibrosis transmembrane regulator (CFTR) gene. CFTR gene mutation leads to unregulated secretions in the airways resulting in high viscosity in the lungs, favoring pulmonary infection and inflammation during neutrophil recruitment. Neutrophils have been shown to release large amounts of nuclear

NETosis. DOI: https://doi.org/10.1016/B978-0-12-816147-0.00006-X

material through NETosis into the airways of CF patients, which can contribute to the disease pathology. Bactericidal permeability-increasing (BPI) protein is an antimicrobial peptide, which targets Gram-negative bacteria and is stored in azurophilic granules of neutrophils. It becomes localized into NET following PMA-induced NET formation. CF patients develop anti-BPI autoantibodies, levels of which negatively correlate with lung function (Skopelja et al., 2016). This gives further evidence that NETs are involved in autoimmunity in CF. Further, some studies suggested that the extracellular DNA levels associate with neutrophil counts and can be used as a parameter to determine the inflammation and lung disease severity. NET generation can contribute to airway colonization by bacteria, since they are the most frequently found microorganisms in CF patients.

Recent investigations revealed that NET formation promotes mucus thickening in the patient's alveoli and causes it to become sticky, allowing the bacterial colonization of *Haemophilus influenzae*, *Staphylococcus aureus*, and *Pseudomonas aeruginosa* specifically (Manzenreiter et al., 2012). Bacterial colonization can promote neutrophils infiltration that undergoes NETosis, increasing the viscosity of the sputum and consequently lowering the respiratory capacity of CF patients.

Reports suggest that the amount of free DNA is plentiful in the sputum of CF patients, with weakened lung function showing that the airway hindrance is because of the build-up of NET DNA (Dubois et al., 2012; Dwyer et al., 2014; Marcos et al., 2015; Papayannopoulos, Staab, & Zychlinsky, 2011). Moreover it has been reported that the components of NET [i.e., neutrophil elastase (NE), MPO, and histones] can induce destruction of epithelial, endothelial, and connective tissues further deteriorating the lung pathology (Klebanoff, Kinsella, & Wight, 1993; Manzenreiter et al., 2012; Saffarzadeh et al., 2012). The importance of NET in the CF disorder is undermined by insights depicting that removal of free DNA from patient's air route establish a vital treatment for battling CF patients since the administration of recombinant human DNase (rhDNase) yields a significant change in the patient's health (Rahman & Gadjeva, 2014).

Despite the fact that NET carries a collection of weaponry to sequester and impair the spread of bacteria, they fare better at trapping than killing. NET-mediated immunity depends on the mechanical clearance from the mucosal surfaces, and, when this fails, in cases such as CF, NET may drive bacterial micro colonization. In this sense, the utilization of DNase I, once bacteria have colonized the lungs, will not be sufficient as when administered much earlier to prevent colonization. Alternatively novel ways to regulate NETosis should be discovered to restrain prolific extracellular DNA presence and the resulting inflammatory responses. Treatment for CF patients is the administration of rhDNase to disrupt the NET structure and so liquefy the sputum and facilitate mucociliary clearance (Papayannopoulos et al., 2011).

Antimicrobial role of neutrophil extracellular trap in cystic fibrosis

NETs have been conserved throughout evolution for their antimicrobial role. CFTR neutrophils have impaired antimicrobial capacity and abnormal variations in the pH of their cytoplasm, dysregulated protein trafficking, excessive NE, and myeloperoxidase (MPO) function, and diminished hypochlorite concentrations in their phagolysosomes. Furthermore neutrophils from CF patients have less intrinsic apoptosis and may be therefore more likely to make NET. CFTR macrophages have high intraphagolysosomal pH and increased Toll-like receptor 4 on their cell surface membranes, which inhibit their antimicrobial capacity and render them hyperresponsive to inflammatory stimuli, respectively (Law & Gray, 2017).

According to studies in humans it was described that NET has antimicrobial properties, although laboratory strains and CF clinical isolates of *P. aeruginosa* strongly trigger NET discharge (Rada, 2017), late isolates within CF airways procure obstruction against NET (Martínez-Alemán et al., 2017; Young et al., 2011). Fuchs et al. (2007) demonstrated that only 25% of neutrophils form NET to kill *S. aureus* in vitro; the majority of bacterial killing occurs by phagocytosis. NETosis appears better suited to tackling large microbes, such as fungal hyphae, which are too large to be phagocytosed (Branzk et al., 2014). Marcos et al. (2015) reported that NET in air route tests of CF patients were found to associate with contagious colonization of *Aspergillus fumigatus* but not with bacterial contamination. So it is hypothesized in regard to CF that NET could play only a minor antimicrobial role, as regardless of the presence of large numbers of activated neutrophils and extracellular DNA, patients suffer current lower respiratory tract infections and colonization with organisms such as *S. aureus*, *P. aeruginosa*, and *A. fumigates* as the host's defense mechanisms are overwhelmed. On one hand, fulfill their bacteriostatic and bactericidal roles in lower order species effectively (Kenny et al., 2017) but on the other hand, due to the presence of an adaptive innate immune system, function as detrimental autoantigens in human autoimmune disease.

Pathophysiological role of neutrophil extracellular trap in cystic fibrosis

NET formation can be activated by *P. aeruginosa* (Yoo, Floyd, Winn, Moskowitz, & Rada, 2014), a major pathogen in CF lung disease, and several studies have shown that NET level is elevated in airway samples from CF patients compared to healthy controls and are associated with poorer lung function (Dwyer et al., 2014; Marcos et al., 2015). DNase is a treatment primarily administered in adult CF patients and it is speculated that it targets NET DNA. It is a nebulized treatment used to enhance patients' lung function and reduce exacerbation rate in both pediatric and adult patients (Fuchs et al., 1994; Hubbard et al., 1992; Quan et al., 2001). It has the capacity to cleave the excessive extracellular DNA to diminish sputum thickness (Lieberman, 1968) and it additionally decreases airway inflammation (Konstan & Ratjen, 2012). This DNA spine of NET is the platform whereupon a few proinflammatory proteins belonging to this process such as histones, NE, calprotectin, and BPI bind.

Alternative fates of neutrophils in the cystic fibrosis lung

In the normal course in the lung, neutrophils encounter and phagocytose bacteria. Following phagocytosis neutrophils rapidly undergo apoptosis and clearance by macrophages thus promoting resolution of inflammation. Alternatively the excess of bacteria in the CF airway may lead to neutrophils forming NET in addition to normal phagocytosis. NET may contribute to host defense, but also allow the release of toxic components into the airway that can damage the host lung. We can postulate that NET contributes to the failed resolution of inflammation in the CF lung, and the clearance of NET by macrophages may not be as antiinflammatory as the clearance of apoptotic neutrophils (Gray, McCullagh, & McCray, 2015).

Neutrophil extracellular trap−based therapeutic options in cystic fibrosis

Presence of high levels of extracellular DNA is the hallmark of CF. Traditionally extracellular DNA was seen to be originating from cellular debris. One well-known symptomatic choice of treatment for CF is the rhDNase I (rhDNAse/Pulmozyme/dornase alfa) (Konstan et al., 2011) to clear the unusually elevated amounts of extracellular DNA present (Papayannopoulos et al., 2011). Clinical proof demonstrates that treatment with Dornase alfa over a constrained timeframe running from 1 to 2 years can result in moderate improvement of lung function. Most of the Dornase alfa preliminaries incorporate patients with age range from childhood to adulthood. This makes it hard to assess whether there is a particular treatment where the rhDNase I is most helpful to patients. Treatment with rhDNase Pulmozyme has also been shown to lead to a decrease in the concentration and length of extracellular DNA in CF (Brandt, Breitenstein, von der Hardt, & Tummler, 1995). Some authors suggest that a complex association of extracellular DNA, NE, and MPO exists in CF sputum and solubilization of sputum relied upon NET-discharged elastase that proteolytically targeted NET-related histones (Papayannopoulos et al., 2011). It has been shown time and again that it is most likely that the majority of the extracellular DNA is NET derived, this indicates toward an intensified innate immune response that fails to target the bacterial colonizer while allowing for the inflammatory milieu leading to pathoadaptation of bacteria that can partially contribute to the etiology of CF symptoms. All these studies clearly indicate that NET is responsible for bacterial maintenance, and, henceforth, advance bacterial colonization, where early treatment with rhDNAse might be more valuable than late in evading further complications. CF patients are prevalently colonized with *P. aeruginosa* species. It is suspected that this happens due to the debilitated mucociliary transport considering the chronical microbial disease without mechanical clearance.

With our present insight of NET biology, some concern exists with respect to the utilization of DNase I specifically due to the tendency of DNase I to discharge NET-resident elastase, which subsequently degrades histones (Papayannopoulos et al., 2011). Since histones are a part of NET that facilitates bacterial adhesion and sequestration, histone reduction may yield diminishing bacterial sequestration. If bacteria were not adequately killed by NET, due to DNase I treatment it might contribute to the release of pathogenic microbes and exacerbation of infection, to a limited extent in the CF patients. One approach to address this entanglement is the use of an elastase inhibitor alongside DNase I, another way is diminishing the NETosis procedure by inhibiting an upstream molecule. There are other methods and drugs to diminish NETosis, for example, chloroquine, an antimalarial drug that inhibits NET generation. PAD4 inhibitors correspondingly diminish NETosis. Another potential way to deal with controlling NET discharge is the Siglec 9 neutrophil surface receptor.

NE enhances solubilization of sputum by degrading histones and facilitating the access for rhDNase. NET and their modulating enzymes such as lysozyme and proteases, antimicrobial peptides (BPI protein and defensins), ion chelators, and histones are able to kill the pathogens. On the other hand the liberated elastase, as well as other proteolytic NET components can damage lung tissues and enhance the immune response by modulating the inflammatory factors, for example, active proteases can degrade surfactant protein D (SP-D), during pathogenic infection. However, NE in CF sputum is predominantly bound to DNA, which downregulates its proteolytic activity but also precludes the inhibition by exogenous protease inhibitors (Dubois et al., 2012). Considering the benefits and problems resulting from the mucolytic therapy, it seems reasonable to introduce a combination therapy with rhDNase and protease inhibitors, which should offer the best compromise between lung tissue injury and easy mucus removal (Zawrotniak & Rapala-Kozik, 2013).

NETosis in diabetes mellitus

Diabetes mellitus (DM) is the most important metabolic disease posing a significant global threat to public health. Symptoms are premature death, disability, and several other complications. The prevalence of DM is steadily rising in developing and developed countries reaching the epidemic status. The progression of this disease relates to developing vasculopathies, for example, retinopathy, micro-, and macroangiopathies, which adversely affect the clinical outcome as well as worsen the quality of life.

As compared to the controlled population the risk of vasculopathies in DM patients is 2−4 times higher. However, these DM-induced vasculopathies are associated with type 1 DM (T1DM) and type 2 DM (T2DM) and do not closely relate to chronic hyperglycemia represented by glycated hemoglobin and glycemic variability (Caprnda et al., 2017; Tong, Chi, & Zhang, 2018). Developing vasculopathy in DM associates with early atherosclerosis, stroke, unstable angina/myocardial infarction, blinding, advanced limb ischemia, nephropathy, and thrombotic complications (Kakuta et al., 2017; Medical Advisory Secretariat, 2010; Wei et al., 2016). Moreover the risk of death due to vascular impurities dramatically rises as high as up to eightfold in DM patients in comparison with those who had none of these complications (Mohammedi et al., 2016). It was well established that vasculopathy in DM results in various other complications, such as exaggerated oxidative stress, impaired vascular repair, endothelial dysfunction, systemic and microvascular inflammation, acceleration of atherosclerosis due to fluctuated hyperglycemia, and remarkable lipotoxicity (Lehoux & Jones, 2016).

The common factor that triggers vasculopathy in different types of DM is microvascular inflammation, which corresponds to metabolic abnormalities and is under tight control of (epi)-genetic regulation and immune/antigen-presenting cells (Yamagishi, Nakamura, Suematsu, Kaseda, & Matsui, 2015). Hyperglycemia, metabolic abnormalities, oxidative stress components (reactive oxygen species, advanced glycation end-products), chemokines, cellular adhesive molecule, hormones (endothelin-1, aldosterone, angiotensin-II) interact with neutrophils and macrophages via several intercellular signaling pathways (i.e., PI3K/Akt/eNOs/NF-kB and ERK1/2/p38 MAPK-activated protein kinases), and recruit predominantly neutrophil subsets in the vasculature promoting inflammation through not just synthesis and releasing of proinflammatory cytokines (TNF-α, IL-2, IL-8, adiponectin, vistafin), but shaping of NET (Leavy, 2015). Despite the fact that there are striking contrasts in the prevalence of vasculopathy in different types of DM, hyperglycemia and lipotoxicity are considered as major factors contributing to vascular complications through inducing NET. NET has been suggested as a link between endothelium, aggravation, and thrombosis that is critical for improvement of DM-prompted vasculopathy. It has been recommended that NET formation could be an objective for the DM care, as well as a biomarker for stratification of DM patients.

Previous studies have demonstrated that the neutrophils isolated from peripheral blood of diabetics showed spontaneous NETosis and NET

(Berezin, 2016a, 2016b, 2016c). Hyperglycemia exhibited NET-inducing capacity associated with elevated levels of circulating markers of NETosis including free cell DNA, elastase, mono-, and oligonucleosomes (Fadini, Menegazzo, Rigato et al., 2016; Fadini, Menegazzo, Scattolini, et al., 2016). Indeed basal levels of NET in T2DM patients were higher compared to healthy volunteers and related to fasting hyperglycemia, an attenuation of glycemia status with metformin was not totally connected with the suppressed activity of TNF-α- and PMA-induced NETosis. According to reports hyperglycemia was controlled in 6 months of metformin treatment, although basal level and stimulated form of NETosis showed normal values in 12 months together with circulating biomarkers of NETosis, such as IL-6, TNF-α, cell-free DNAs (Carestia et al., 2016). Joshi et al. (2016) have reported the formation of NETosis in neutrophils exposed to high glucose level, homocysteine, and IL-6. Hyperglycemic condition is closely related to homocysteine, but homocysteine triggers NETosis via NADPH oxidase−dependent and −independent mechanisms in a glucose interdependent manner. Thus it has been suggested that increased level of NETosis in T2DM patients did not impair glycemic control rather is related to inflammation. In this specific circumstance, unconstrained and inducible NETosis in DM may correlate with various molecular pathways.

NETosis severely impairs wound healing in diabetes mellitus

Wound healing is disabled in diabetes resulting in significant high rate of morbidity and mortality. Neutrophils are the fundamental leukocytes associated with the early phase of healing. Expression of peptidylarginine deiminase 4 (PAD4), an enzyme important in chromatin decondensation, and mediating NETosis is upregulated in individuals with diabetes as compared to healthy controls. Under diabetic conditions, neutrophils produce more superoxide (Karima et al., 2005) and cytokines (Hanses, Park, Rich, & Lee, 2011). TNF-α, a proinflammatory cytokine, involved in NETosis is increased in diabetic individuals (Alexandraki et al., 2008).

Circulating NET-related biomarkers, nucleosomes, cell-free double-stranded DNA, and NE are increased in the sera of individuals with type 2 diabetes, and nucleosomes positively correlate with these individuals' HbA1c levels (Menegazzo et al., 2015). A high concentration of NE can cause degradation of the wound matrix and delay healing (Herrick et al., 1997). Because PAD4 is not expressed in the skin, its negative effect on wound healing is most likely due to infiltrating neutrophils (Nachat et al., 2005). *Staphylococcus* species are very abundant in diabetic wounds and degrade NET DNA to escape trapping (Berends et al., 2010) hence, using NETosis to defend against microbes may not be very effective during wound healing. Wound healing could be similarly affected in individuals with decreased DNase I activity.

Antineutrophil extracellular trap therapy in diabetes mellitus

As DNase I cleaves NET to enhance wound recovery; it is an effective inhibitor of PAD4, which is overproduced by activated neutrophils in diabetic individuals. It could be a novel therapeutic approach to wound healing in diabetes as well as to other diseases such as normoglycemic patients. The increased NETosis in diabetes suggests that it may fuel these disorders and inhibit NETosis or cleavage may lessen them.

Metformin treatment reduced the concentrations of NET components independently from glucose control. This effect was reproducible in vitro and was related to the inhibitory effect exerted by metformin on the PKC-NADPH oxidase pathway. This NET inhibiting pharmacologic effect of metformin can potentially improve immune-inflammation in DM (Menegazzo et al., 2015).

NETosis in cardiometabolic disease

Cardiovascular disorder is the leading cause of morbidity and mortality in diabetic patients. Activated macrophages, the role of which in the pathogenesis of atherosclerosis and peripheral artery disease is now well established could maintain inducible NETosis of neutrophils in T2DM and thereby contribute in accelerating atherosclerosis (Menegazzo et al., 2015; Sollberger, Tilley, & Zychlinsky, 2018). Various other stimuli, that is, ischemia/hypoxia, oxidized lipoproteins, free unsaturated fats, necrotic cells, and modified histones, might be triggers for neutrophils to release NET via an endogenous danger signal, which are able to activate stress-responsive transcription factor, Nrf2, and regulate synthesis of inflammasome with proinflammatory cytokines (IL-1α and IL-1β) (Freigang et al., 2013; Menegazzo et al., 2015; Warnatsch, Ioannou, Wang, & Papayannopoulos, 2015). NETs are essential components of plaques and probably they contribute to the generation of autoantibodies that lead to aggravation of atherosclerotic lesion of the vasculature. There is evidence that atherosclerosis may have been enhanced by augmenting NET formation within the plaque activation of peripheral blood polymorphonuclear myeloid−derived suppressor cells, but not of inflammatory monocytes/macrophages (Freigang et al., 2013; Yamamoto et al., 2018). Interestingly, Pertiwi et al. (2018), have concluded that NETosis could be a prominent pro-thrombotic player in all distinct types of atherosclerosis and thrombosis, which facilitates the progression of vascular complications and thus the onset of ensuing clinical peripheral artery ischemic syndromes. Thus the molecular mechanisms of programmed cell death- apoptosis and NETosis connect inflammation and atherosclerosis, by promoting accumulation of pro-atherogenic, thrombotic factors and cell debris in circulation and thus contributing toward progression of the peripheral artery disease. Clinical investigations have demonstrated that elevated levels of serum dsDNA as a marker of NETosis was related to the presence of cardiovascular (CV) sickness, atherosclerosis, nephropathy, peripheral artery disease in patients with T2DM (Fadini, Menegazzo, Rigato et al., 2016; Fadini, Menegazzo, Scattolini, et al., 2016; Mangold et al., 2015). There is evidence that T2DM-induced vasculopathy that showed up before atherosclerotic plaque accumulation and associated with endothelial dysfunction was clearly associated to apoptotic endothelial cell originated chromatin-contained microvesicles, which are triggers for NETosis (Aghajanian, Wittchen, Campbell, & Burridge, 2009; Wang et al., 2012). Furthermore cell-free dsDNA levels associated positively with morphological evidence of plaque destabilization, severity of peripheral artery disease and the risk of limb ischemia, as well as CV mortality rate (Berezin, 2016a, 2016b, 2016c). NETosis in T2DM could probably serve as a biomarker of higher risk of microvascular inflammation, endothelial dysfunction, thrombotic complication, and atherosclerosis (Megens et al., 2012).

Increased peptidylarginine deiminase 4 and neutrophil extracellular trap activation in atherosclerosis

Recently Warnatsch et al. (2015) showed that neutrophils prime macrophages for proinflammatory responses in atherosclerotic plaques. This priming is mediated by NET, extracellular webs of DNA bound to cytotoxic histones, which are released by activated neutrophils (Brinkmann et al., 2004). This process of NET formation follows a coordinated multistep process: histone citrullination, chromatin decondensation, migration of elastase and other granule enzymes into the nucleus, disintegration of the nuclear membrane and release of DNA, histones, and granule proteins into the extracellular space (Fadini, Menegazzo, Rigato et al., 2016; Fadini, Menegazzo, Scattolini, et al., 2016). The release of NET primes macrophages to produce pro-IL-1β, which is cleaved to mature proinflammatory IL-1β by caspase 1. Caspase 1, in turn, is secreted by macrophages in response to activation of the NLRP3 (NOD-like receptor family, pyrin domain-containing 3) inflammasome. NET is also pro-thrombotic (Warnatsch et al., 2015). Neutrophils from type 1 and type 2 diabetic humans as well as mice are primed to produce NET and have increased expression of PAD4. Increased PAD4 transcription is driven by NFκB, which is chronically activated in diabetes. Hyperglycemia-induced ROS likely activate PAD4 as well, by increasing intracellular Ca^{2+} concentration. Other consequences of increased intracellular ROS such as PKC activation increase levels of the NET-priming cytokine TNF-α. Normal resolution of inflammation caused by infiltration of neutrophils and macrophages involves a switch from synthesis of arachidonic acid−derived prostaglandins and leukotrienes to synthesis of lipoxins, which stop neutrophil recruitment.

NETosis-based therapy

There is not much indication of the potential of anti-NET therapy in arthero-sclerosis and cardiometabolic disease. Studies to determine whether anti-NET/antiinflammatory therapies can improve cardiovascular outcomes are necessary before these treatments become a part of cardiovascular prevention.

NETosis in cancer

Cancer remains a devastating cause of mortality worldwide, with the majority of patients dying as a result of metastasis (Kumar & Sharma, 2010; Lip, Chin, & Blann, 2002; Sica, Schioppa, Mantovani, & Allavena, 2006). Novel data indicate that neutrophil function is modified in a malignant disease. Neutrophils may become prominent disease promoters, contributing to angiogenesis and metastasis during tumor progression (Gregory & Houghton, 2011). NET was detected in individuals with cancer for the first time a few years ago (Berger-Achituv et al., 2013; Demers et al., 2012), and the consequences are only beginning to emerge. Based on several reports it is now convincing to believe that immune cells have a major impact on cancer development and progression. The role of both platelets and neutrophils as autonomous regulators of various processes in cancer has been known for long, however, it has quite recently emerged that the platelet–neutrophil interplay is yet a critical component to take into account during malignant disease. It was reported that neutrophils in mice with cancer have an increased tendency to form NET-like structure by chromatin and secreted proteases. Moreover the presence of NET in humans with cancer has been confirmed in a few recent investigations, showing that tumor-induced NET is clinically applicable (Olsson & Cedervall, 2016). A few reports have also suggested that NET contribute to cancer-associated pathology by promoting processes responsible for cancer-related death such as thrombosis, systemic inflammation, and relapse of the disease. It has been demonstrated that platelets can act as inducers of intravascular NETosis in response to lipopolysaccharide (LPS) (Clark et al., 2007; Jenne, Urrutia, & Kubes, 2013). Conversely NET provides a strong activation signal for platelets due to the externalized DNA and associated histones, promoting platelet aggregation and thrombosis (Fuchs et al., 2010). The platelet–neutrophil interface can be an important component to consider when designing therapies targeting cancer-associated pathology in the future.

The occurrence of cancer is commonly associated with the manifestation of a variety of clinical thrombotic syndromes including local and systemic venous and arterial thromboses (Gregory & Houghton, 2011; Kumar & Sharma, 2010). In fact thrombosis is frequently associated with a worse prognosis of neoplastic disease as it is often diagnosed as the first clinical manifestation of a tumor. Despite a large number of epidemiological studies investigating the incidence, prevalence, and treatment of thrombosis in cancer patients, the mechanisms underlying the pathogenesis of this process have not been completely elucidated. Increased leukocyte amount is a well-known predictor of cancer-associated thrombosis (Cortjens et al., 2016; Urban, Reichard, Brinkmann, & Zychlinsky, 2006). Recent studies have shown that neutrophils play a major role in arterial (Bruns et al., 2010) and venous (Springer et al., 2010) thrombus development. The involvement of neutrophils in thrombus formation is dependent on the formation of NET, which is described as web-like structures of DNA and proteins formed through a process called NETosis. The negatively charged surface of NET results in the activation of contact phase proteins such as FXII. In addition, NET activates platelets and inactivate local endogenous anticoagulants. (Bianchi, Niemiec, Siler, Urban, & Reichenbach, 2011; Gazendam et al., 2016). Therefore DNase I mediated disruption of NETosis is a treatment which can be utilized in arresting the development of thrombosis. Remarkably, tumor cell−derived exosomes induce NET formation in neutrophils from granulocyte colony-stimulating factor (G-CSF)−treated mice and accelerate venous thrombus formation in tumor-free neutrophilic mice. Our observations suggest that tumor-associated neutrophilia and tendency to the NET formation is associated with increased levels of G-CSF (Demers et al., 2012; Warnatsch et al., 2015; Wong et al., 2015). Treatment with tumor-derived exosomes triggers NET formation in neutrophils of G-CSF-treated mice and accelerate venous thrombus formation in tumor-free neutrophilic mice (Demers et al., 2012). It is suggested that tumor-derived exosomes and neutrophils act synergistically in the establishment of cancer-associated thrombosis.

Consequences of neutrophil extracellular trap in cancer

Tumor-induced NET may be a promoter of cancer-associated pathology. For instance Cools-Lartigue and colleagues (2013) demonstrated that infection-induced NET contributes to metastasis by sequestration of tumor cells in the circulation of mice with cancer. This suggests an increased risk for metastasis if cancer patients are affected by an infectious disease. Besides the direct impact on malignant progression, tumor-induced NETosis additionally contributes to systemic pathological effects of cancer. As NET has been shown to promote cancer-associated deep vein thrombosis (Berger-Achituv et al., 2013), the procoagulant effect of NET is primarily mediated through the negatively charged DNA initiating the intrinsic pathway of coagulation (Gould et al., 2014) and by histones contributing to thrombin formation (Ammollo, Semeraro, Xu, Esmon, & Esmon, 2011). TF and factor XII, both inducers of the extrinsic and intrinsic coagulation pathways, respectively can be found in NET (Kambas et al., 2012; Kambas et al., 2013; von Brühl et al., 2012).

Therapeutic targeting of neutrophil extracellular trap in individuals with cancer

The role of tumor-induced NET as potential promoters of malignancy and associated complications, such as thrombosis and systemic inflammation, suggests that therapeutic approaches to suppress NET might be beneficial for cancer patients. Several potential strategies could be considered. Strategy to degrade extracellular DNA strands through treatment with DNase I, would be an option to disintegrate NET. As discussed previously DNase I and PAD4 inhibitors are already known for the treatment of patients with CF, DM, etc., which indicates their safety as a drug (Tomson, 1995). In addition, a third alternative method would be treatment with heparin, which has a capacity to destabilize NET by extraction of histones (Fuchs et al., 2010). Heparin has an anticoagulative capacity well known for a long time and also has been established as a reasonably successful therapeutic approach. Based on the current information (Olsson & Cedervall, 2016), NET induction associated with the P-selectin (on activated platelets/PSGL-1 (on neutrophils) interaction could present them as potential therapeutic targets (Fig. 6.1). Further research is necessary to fully explore the potential risks associated with therapeutic approaches targeting NET. The current information on tumor-induced NET strongly indicates that targeting NET could be beneficial

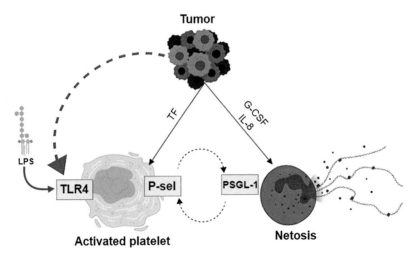

FIGURE 6.1 Platelet–neutrophil crosstalk in tumor-induced NETosis. Tumor cells can directly induce NETosis by secretion of factors such as G-CSF and IL-8. It may further promote platelet activation by production of tissue factor (TF). Activated platelets act as NETosis inducers. This effect is mediated via direct binding of P-selectin on activated platelets and PSGL-1 on neutrophils. Stimulation of platelets via Toll-like receptor 4 (TLR4) by lipopolysaccharide (LPS) during infectious disease or tumor-derived factors may further contribute to platelet-induced NETosis.

for cancer patients. NET, initially recognized as a defense mechanism against severe infectious disease, seem rather to have a negative influence during malignant disease by promoting mortal processes such as thrombosis, systemic inflammation, and cancer relapse. Considering this, NET could provide future anticancer drug targets, with the capacity to suppress processes leading to cancer-related deaths.

Neutrophil extracellular trap in Alzheimer's disease

AD is a neurodegenerative disorder characterized by the progressive deterioration of cognitive functions. Its neuropathology is characterized by amyloid-β (Aβ) accumulation, the development of neurofibrillary tangles, and the loss of neurons and synapses. The primary neuropathological features of AD include neuritic plaques formed by deposits of amyloid-β (Aβ), the abnormal accumulation of hyperphosphorylated tau protein in the neuronal soma, as neurofibrillary tangles (NFTs), synaptic dysfunction, and neuronal loss (Querfurth & LaFerla, 2010). Additionally, AD is also characterized by cerebral amyloid angiopathy due to Aβ deposits in the cerebral vasculature, which cause luminal stenosis, endothelial damage, basement membrane thickening, thrombosis, loss of autoregulation, and vasospasm (Love, 2010).

Evidence strongly suggests that AD-related inflammation develops in the blood and the brain both of which are two interrelated compartments. In this perspective systemic inflammation can lead to "brain activation," whereas cerebral inflammation may influence the peripheral system through the release of danger signals and other inflammatory molecules (Abbott, Rönnbäck, & Hansson, 2006; Heneka et al., 2015; Zlokovic, 2011; Zenaro, Piacentino, & Constantin, 2017). Recently NET has been reported to be observed within the cerebral vasculature and parenchyma of animal AD models and individuals with AD, proposing that NET can potentially harm the blood−brain barrier (BBB) and neural cells (Zenaro et al., 2015).

During pathogenesis of several neuroinflammatory disorders a central process that manifests itself is the recruitment of neutrophils from the CNS. It ranges from bacterial and viral encephalitis to noninfectious conditions, such as cerebral ischemia, trauma, and demyelinating syndromes (Holmin, Söderlund, Biberfeld, & Mathiesen, 1998; Kenne, Erlandsson, Lindbom, Hillered, & Clausen, 2012; Miller, Wang, Tan, & Dittel, 2015; Rossi, Angiari, Zenaro, Budui, & Constantin, 2011). Previous studies have demonstrated that neutrophils transmigration in the CNS obtain a toxic phenotype and approach neuronal cells, where they release harmful molecules and can compromise neuronal functions (Allen et al., 2012). Therefore limiting neutrophil migration and/or functions can positively influence the outcome of neuronal injuries (Kenne et al., 2012; Miller et al., 2015; Zenaro et al., 2015, 2017).

Two types of NETosis in Alzheimer's disease: intravascular and intraparenchymal NET

Intravascular NETosis

Intravascular NET simply refers to its induction within a blood vessel or blood vascular system. The release of intravascular NET by adherent neutrophils has been observed in several diseases, including sepsis, atherosclerosis, autoimmune pathologies, such as autoimmune small-vessel vasculitis, experimental deep vein thrombosis, transfusion-related acute lung injury, and cancer. It can be triggered by different stimuli including microbes, antibody−antigen complexes, proinflammatory cytokines, and activated platelets (Fig. 6.2).

Accordingly, in vitro studies suggest that Aβ peptides could play an important role in the endothelial activation and intravascular neutrophil adhesion in AD (Giri et al., 2000; Zenaro et al., 2015). Recent studies indicate that both oligomeric and fibrillary Aβ1−42 trigger the rapid, integrin-dependent adhesion of human and mouse neutrophils on fibrinogen and ICAM-1, a ligand for LFA-1 integrin (Zenaro et al., 2015). Additionally, Aβ1−42 has been shown to induce both the intermediate-affinity and high-affinity states of LFA-1, potentially providing stop signals for neutrophils.

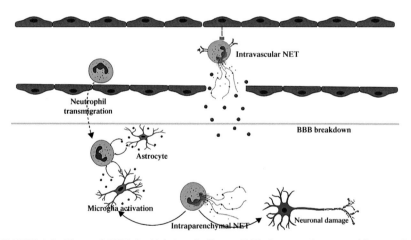

FIGURE 6.2 **Types of NETs in Alzheimer's disease (AD).** Intravascular neutrophil extracellular traps (NETs) potentially produced by the contribution of activated platelets probably through the binding of neutrophil LFA-1 with platelet ICAM-2. Extracellular DNA and components such as histones, myeloperoxidase (MPO), neutrophil elastase, and cathepsin G, released during NET formation, induce the production of proinflammatory cytokines and thrombin, contributing to the loss of blood−brain barrier integrity. Neutrophils present inside the cerebral parenchyma are activated by inflammatory mediators released by glial cells and produce NETs, which may further activate glial cells and damage surrounding neurons. NETs contribute toward neutrophil-mediated intravascular and intraparenchymal tissue damage in AD.

Furthermore it is recognized that intravascular neutrophil adhesion and the release of NET in the human brains affected by AD, suggesting that intravascular NET may also contribute to CNS damage in humans. The cerebral vasculature in AD subjects is strongly activated and produces cytokines, suggesting that intravascular cytokines may favor the formation of NET in this context.

AD brain microvessels release significantly higher levels of thrombin, TNF-α, IL-1β, and IL-8 than age-matched controls, indicating that such endothelial molecules may promote the formation of NET by adherent neutrophils (Grammas & Ovase, 2001; Grammas, Samany, & Tirumangalakudi, 2006; Yin, Wright, Wall, & Grammas, 2010). Thrombin becomes more abundant in the cerebral capillaries of AD brains and induces the release of IL-1β and IL-8, which may in turn contribute to intravascular NETosis (Grammas, Samany, & Tirumangalakudi, 2006; Keshari et al., 2012; Pillitteri et al., 2007; Ueno, Murakami, Yamanouchi, Watanabe, & Kondo, 1996; Yin et al., 2010). Interestingly subjects with mild cognitive impairment have higher serum IL-1β levels than controls, suggesting this cytokine may trigger the release of NET and contribute to the onset of AD (Forlenza et al., 2009). In vitro investigations of brain endothelial cells have shown that the expression of cytokine genes including IL-1β, were increased by Aβ peptides, which trigger NETosis (Vukic et al., 2009)

Intraparenchymal NETosis

Neutrophils invade the brain parenchyma of AD mouse models at the early stage of AD and contribute to the induction of memory deficit (Pietronigro, Della Bianca, Zenaro, & Constantin, 2017). Neutrophils migrating to intraparenchymal regions produce NET, indicating that cells releasing MPO, NE, and citrullinated histone H3 are present in the parenchyma of AD mouse models. During AD intraparenchymal cytokines, such as TNF-α, IL-1β, and IL-8, produced by neural cells may also promote NET formation in extravasated neutrophils (Keshari et al., 2012). Accordingly, activated astrocytes and microglia in AD patients secrete proinflammatory cytokines, such as IL-1β, TNF-α, and IL-8, as well as ROS into the surrounding brain tissue rich in Aβ deposits, thus potentially contributing to intraparenchymal NET formation and generating crosstalk with intraparenchymal neutrophils (Fig. 6.2.) (Czirr & Wyss-Coray, 2012; Heneka et al., 2015; Heppner, Ransohoff, & Becher, 2015). Immunohistochemistry studies have shown that neutrophils migrate inside the parenchymal areas containing Aβ plaques and less neuronal fluorescence, indicating that Aβ may have a role in the migration of neutrophils inside the parenchyma and in providing stop signals for neutrophils. Aβ triggers ROS generation by activating NADPH oxidase in vitro in both human and mouse neutrophils and, ROS production is crucial to the formation of NET (Pietronigro et al., 2017). These data support for the role of Aβ in the intraparenchymal NET formation and neutrophil-dependent CNS damage during AD.

Recent findings show that both TNF-α and IL-1β have a role in NETosis associated with rheumatoid arthritis and gout, suggesting that there are chances they may contribute to the NET formation in AD patients as well (Khandpur et al., 2013; Mitroulis et al., 2011). Furthermore treatment with anakinra (a recombinant IL-1 receptor antagonist) or a monoclonal antibody that blocks IL-1β caused the partial inhibition of NET in gout (Mitroulis et al., 2011). Higher levels of IL-1β and TNF-α are found in the brain and cerebrospinal fluid (CSF) of AD patients, suggesting they may contribute to neutrophil activation and NET formation in AD (Griffin et al., 1989; Tarkowski, Andreasen, Tarkowski, & Blennow, 2003). Furthermore recent studies show that IL-17 contributes to NETosis in rheumatoid arthritis and in a model of acute myocardial infarction, suggesting that this cytokine may favor NET formation also in AD (de Boer et al., 2013; Khandpur et al., 2013). These combined data suggest that proinflammatory cytokines may act in concert with Aβ and ROS to promote intraparenchymal NETosis in AD.

During the generation of NET the azurophilic granules of neutrophils release MMPs, specifically MMP-9, and serine proteases such as NE, cathepsin G, and MPO, which can induce tissue damage and aggravate the inflammatory process. MMPs are involved in the proteolysis of the extracellular matrix and can thus damage the brain parenchyma. NE can induce the degradation of tissues by activating MMPs and inactivating the endogenous tissue inhibitors of MMPs (TIMPs) (Itoh & Nagase, 1995). Furthermore inhibition of MMP-9 that is expressed in senile plaques, NET, and the vascular walls of human AD brains may be therapeutic targets for AD patients.

Neutrophil extracellular trap−based therapeutic approaches in Alzheimer's disease

NETosis inhibition has yielded therapeutic benefits in several models of inflammatory diseases, including autoimmune diseases affecting the brain. Therefore targeting of NET may delay AD pathogenesis and offer a novel approach for the treatment of AD. However, the effect of blocking NET formation in AD animal models has not yet been demonstrated and further studies are required to determine whether this approach has merit. Inhibition of neutrophil trafficking may also be beneficial in AD.

In conclusion NET represents a novel disease mechanism in AD and targeting their effects during sterile inflammation may provide an additional therapeutic strategy for the treatment of this devastating disease.

NETosis in gout

Gout is a chronic disease marked by deposition of monosodium urate (MSU) crystals, resulting from increased urate concentrations. At higher levels uric acid crystallizes and the crystals deposit in the joints, tendons, and surrounding tissues, resulting in an attack of gout. Both environmental factors such as hyperuricemia, renal and gut excretion of urate, and genetic factors play an important role in the regulation of serum urate. The release of interleukin 1β plays a key role in the initiation of gout disease. Gout is a common and treatable form of inflammatory arthritis and occurs more commonly in those who regularly eat meat or are overweight. Diagnosis of gout may be confirmed by the presence of crystals in the fluids or in the deposits outside the joint. The clinical features of gout result due to the inflammatory response to MSU crystals and treatment strategies that achieve crystal dissolution are central to the effective gout management. (Khanna et al., 2012). In the last few years, major progress has been made in the understanding of the pathogenesis, impact, diagnostic approaches to, and treatment of this disorder.

Immunology of the acute inflammatory response in gout

A few people with intra-articular depositions of MSU crystals develop an acute inflammatory response, as acute gout flares when MSU crystals interact with resident macrophages to form and activate the "NOD-, LRR- and pyrin domain-containing 3" (NLRP3) inflammasome (Martinon, Petrilli, Mayor, Tardivel, & Tschopp, 2006). This process is facilitated by microtubule-driven spatial colocalization with mitochondria, involving α-tubulin acetylation (Misawa et al., 2013) by the activated inflammasome recruits caspase 1, which converts pro-interleukin 1β into mature interleukin 1β (Martinon et al., 2006). Activated neutrophils and mast cells amplify the inflammatory response, leading to the release of a host of proinflammatory cytokines, chemokines, and other factors such as reactive oxygen species, prostaglandin E2, and lysosomal enzymes (Cronstein & Sunkureddi, 2013). Resolution phase of acute gouty inflammation and induction of anti-inflammatory cytokines and lipid mediators is mediated by aggregated NET structures.

MSU crystals induce neutrophil extracellular trap via a distinct molecular pathway

MSU and other physiologically relevant crystals induce NET through a molecular pathway. Taken together, two essential molecular phases can be distinguished in gout. The first phase is the precipitation of MSU crystals and their ingestion by mononuclear phagocytes leading to inflammasome activation. This molecular process, which depends on the production of

IL-1β and is characterized by the massive recruitment of neutrophils, explains the clinical symptoms of an acute gout attack. The second phase is the formation of tophi resembling aggregated NET, which depends on high densities of neutrophils, and their death by NET formation. The expulsion of DNA during NET densely packs MSU crystals and the formation of aggregated NET neutralizes and degrades the involved proinflammatory cytokines and resolving inflammation (Fig. 6.3) (Chatfield et al., 2018). This molecular process explains the mechanism and clinical picture of chronic tophaceous gout.

Pseudogout and necroptosis induction

Deposition of calcium-containing crystals, calcium pyrophosphate dihydrate (CPP) and basic calcium phosphate (BCP) crystals in the joints and/or soft tissues can result in a variety of articular and periarticular disorders. The clinical manifestation of CPP crystal deposition is known as pseudogout. A robust NET formation of human neutrophils in vitro in response to CPPD crystals has been observed (Pang et al., 2013). In fact CPPD crystals provide a much stronger trigger for NET induction by PMNs than MSU crystals (Pang et al., 2013; Sil et al., 2016) and PMNs phagocytose CPPD crystals are mandatory for CPPD crystal-triggered NET release (Pang et al., 2013).

CPP crystals also induce a regulated form of necrosis (termed necroptosis) in fibroblasts, epithelial cells, and neutrophils (Desai et al., 2017; Mulay et al., 2016). As discussed in earlier chapter necroptosis is associated with the NET formation (Delgado-Rizo et al., 2017). This process occurs independently of caspase activation and probably aggravates tissue injury via the release of additional damage-associated molecular patterns (DAMPs) (Garg et al., 2015). Receptor-interacting serine/threonine-protein kinase 1 (RIPK1), RIPK3 and mixed lineage kinase domain-like protein (MLKL) have important functions in necroptosis and are activated downstream of crystal-induced ROS production (Desai, Mulay, Nakazawa, &

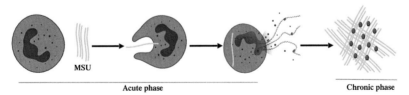

FIGURE 6.3 **NET induction via MSU crystals:** *Acute phase*: Monosodium urate (MSU) crystals uptake by neutrophil phagocytosis leads to release of chemoattractant and induce NETosis. *Chronic Phase*: The expulsion of DNA during neutrophil extracellular trap (NET) densely packs MSU crystals leading to formation of aggregated NETs and the attached proteases neutralize and degrade the involved proinflammatory cytokines thus resolving inflammation.

Anders, 2016). Inhibition of RIPK1 or MLKL with necrostatin 1 and necrosulfonamide, respectively, prevented CPP crystal−induced cell death and associated NET release; hence, the RIPK1−RIPK3−MLKL axis might be a potential therapeutic target to confine necroptosis-associated tissue injury and inflammation in acute CPPD disease (Mitton-Fitzgerald, Gohr, Bettendorf, & Rosenthal, 2016).

Neutrophil extracellular trap−based therapeutic targets in gout

Inhibition of RIPK1 or MLKL with necrostatin 1 and necrosulfonamide, respectively, has shown to prevent CPP crystal−induced cell death and associated NET release; hence, the RIPK1−RIPK3−MLKL axis might be a potential therapeutic target to confine necroptosis-associated tissue injury and inflammation in acute CPPD disease (Mitton-Fitzgerald et al., 2016). Current antiinflammatory gout prophylaxis is limiting and not perfect due to associated potential drug toxicities, drug-drug interactions (Keenan, O'Brien, Lee, Crittenden, Fisher, Goldfarb, Krasnokutsky, Oh, & Pillinger, 2011), and inadequate therapeutic efficacy (Khanna et al., 2012). There is a substantial need for new, and effective antiinflammatory treatment options to prevent and cure gout. Development of novel therapeutics for gout can build upon recently identified host processes that regulate MSU crystal−induced inflammation. NETosis and neutrophil activation serves as a major driver and a resolving component in gout inflammation, as it involves several phagocyte-driven native resolution mechanisms for acute neutrophilic inflammation. These pathways include phagocyte ingestion of apoptotic neutrophils, which leads to an altered profile of inflammatory and antiinflammatory mediators released by effector cells, and NETosis, which also may promote tophus development. New candidates for suppressing gouty inflammation could emerge from targeting modulation of the NET formation.

NETosis in pancreatitis

Acute pancreatitis (AP) refers to inflammation of the pancreas and is typically a mild disease, however, around 20% of the patients develop moderately severe or severe disease (Banks et al., 2013). Moderately severe AP is characterized by the organ dysfunction (OD) and very low mortality (Johnson & Abu-Hilal, 2004) whereas in severe AP, OD is persistent and high mortality, up to 70% is reported (Buter, Imrie, Carter, Evans, & McKay, 2002; Halonen et al., 2002; Johnson & Abu-Hilal, 2004; McKay & Buter, 2003). Studies have suggested that early aggressive intravenous hydration decreases the rate of morbidity and mortality (Tenner, Baillie, DeWitt, & Vege, 2013; Wall et al., 2011). In addition, the patients at risk to develop severe AP, particularly those who present without OD, might benefit from immunomodulatory treatment (Johnson et al., 2001; Kylanpaa et al., 2005; Werner et al., 2012). About half of the AP patients with OD do not have clinical signs of OD at presentation (Johnson et al., 2001; Maksimow et al., 2014; Nieminen et al., 2014). Damaged or dying pancreatic acinar cells release intracellular contents including nuclear DAMPs, such as DNA and histones, which promote the accumulation of innate immune cells into the pancreas and generation of cytokines, among other soluble mediators of inflammation.

It has been proposed that the formation of NET serves to form a transient barrier between necrotic tissues during acute inflammatory processes. NET form in response to necrotic debris and facilitate the clearance of damage-associated molecular patterns (DAMPs) by their binding to the NET. Potentially harmful DAMPs are then degraded in the NET via proteolytic digestion. Extracellular DNA and chromatin-associated proteins then play an important role in coagulation and formation of fibrin clots at the NET surface (Longstaff et al., 2013). Abundant NETosis surrounding necrotic areas in two clinical cases of pancreatitis and peritonitis have been observed.

In acute necrotizing pancreatitis, massive tissue necrosis occurs in and around pancreas resulting in fluid collection organized as pseudocysts. In contrast to regular cysts, these pseudocysts are not surrounded by epithelial layers. It is speculated that the necrotic areas observed in necrotizing pancreatitis are isolated from the surrounding healthy tissues by aggregated NET. These generate an alternative, short-lived barrier, separating necrotic areas from viable tissue. In several affected areas of pancreatic necrosis, NETs were detected by immunohistochemistry and the chromatin was found to be stained positive for NE and citrullinated histone H3. A compact layer of aggregated NET isolates the site of necrosis, thereby limiting the spread of necrosis-associated proinflammatory mediators. The long-term consequences of abundant NET surrounding inflammation areas should be considered, as substantial levels of products of proteolytic digestion are seen in pancreatic pseudocysts (Rojek et al., 2016), and the dying cells have been involved in modulating immune response (Chaurio et al., 2014).

Neutrophil extracellular trap−based therapeutic options in pancreatitis

The ability of NETs to potentially initiate pancreatitis allows for the possibility of therapeutic intervention to prevent excessive neutrophil activation as a treatment option.

A list of molecules with therapeutic potential has been summarized in Table 6.1.

TABLE 6.1 Potential therapeutic molecules for NETosis.

Disease	Molecule	Target	Effects on neutrophils	Effect on disease/clinical use	References
Cystic fibrosis	DNase I (rhDNAse/pulmozyme/dornase alfa)	Excessive extracellular DNA	NET degradation	Improve lung function and reduce exacerbation rate	Quan et al. (2001); Fuchs et al. (1994); Hubbard et al. (1992); Lieberman (1968)
	Protease inhibitor	Regulating the neutrophil elastase activity	NET modulation	Protect the lung, but also lower the neutrophil burden and enhance host defense by protecting complement, complement receptors and locally produced antimicrobials and antiinflammatory molecules	Dubois et al. (2012); Kelly et al. (2008)
Diabetes mellitus	Dnase I	PAD4 inhibition	Cleavage of NET	Wound healing	Wong et al. (2015)
Cardiometabolic disease	PAD4 inhibitor	Deaminates histones (NET contents)	Neutrophils activation	NET-associated pathogenesis	Rohrbach, Hemmers, Arandjelovic, Corr, & Mowen (2012); Wong et al. (2015)
Cancer	DNase or PAD4 inhibitors	PAD4 inhibition	NET inhibition	Prevent tumor spread and cancer-associated thrombosis	Demers & Wagner (2013)

(Continued)

TABLE 6.1 (Continued)

Disease	Molecule	Target	Effects on neutrophils	Effect on disease/clinical use	References
Alzheimer's disease	IL-1β and TNF-α	Activation of NADPH oxidase	Neutrophil activation; intraparenchymal NET formation		Griffin et al. (1989); Tarkowski et al. (2003)
	Anti-LFA-1 integrin	LFA-1 integrin	Blockade of neutrophil trafficking	Disease pathogenesis and cognitive impairment	Zenaro et al. (2015)
Gout	Colchicine	Actin cytoskeleton	Destabilization of NETs or inhibition of NET formation. Improved NET degradation	Used in the management of gout attacks	Neeli, Dwivedi, Khan, and Radic (2009)
	Recombinant IL-1 receptor antagonist (anakinra)	Blocks IL-1β	NET inhibition	Blocks IL-1β caused the partial inhibition of NET formation	Mitroulis et al. (2011)
Pancreatitis	DNase I	Reduced neutrophils infiltration	NET induction		Merza et al. (2015)

NET, neutrophil extracellular trap; PAD4: peptidylarginine deiminase 4.

NETosis in infectious diseases

NETs contain a wide range of antimicrobial factors that kill microbes. The process of NETosis displays effectiveness against a variety of different species of Gram-positive and Gram-negative bacteria, fungi, virus, and parasites and inhibits their growth.

Bacterial diseases

A variety of Gram-negative as well as Gram-positive bacteria has been shown to induce NET formation. Bacterial invasion promotes NET formation which entraps pathogens and obstructs their spread. *S. aureus* is a Gram-positive bacterium and involved in osteomyelitis, endocarditis, bacteremia, and gastroenteritis, which are associated with severe inflammatory response (Liu, 2009). It induces NETosis and escapes host immune system by secretion of numerous virulence factors, such as PVL, leukotoxin GH, leukotoxin DE, gamma-hemolysin, and N-terminal ArgD peptides (Gonzalez, Corriden, Akong-Moore, Olson, Dorrestein, & Nizet, 2014; Malachowa, Kobayashi, Freedman, Dorward, & DeLeo, 2013; Pilsczek, Salina, Poon, Fahey, Yipp, & Sibley, 2015).

Infection with *Streptococcus pneumoniae* leads to community-acquired pneumonia and invasive diseases like meningitis and bacteremia. It is a Gram-positive bacterium having a prominent role in NET induction and promoting spreading of bacteria from upper respiratory tract to the lungs and eventually to the bloodstream (Beiter, Wartha, Albiger, Normark, Zychlinsky, & Henriques-Normark, 2006; Brinkmann et al., 2004; Moorthy, Rai, Jiao, Wang, Tan, & Qin, 2016; Zhu, Kuang, Wilson, & Lau, 2013). Additionally, NET has also been associated with other respiratory diseases resulting from secondary infections such as chronic obstructive pulmonary disease, pneumonia, and emphysema (Bass, Russo, Gabelloni, Geffner, Giordano, & Catalano, 2010; Moorthy et al., 2013; Young et al., 2011).

Escherichia coli, a Gram-negative bacterium that inhabits in the gastrointestinal tract at birth is involved in enteritis, urinary infections, meningitis, and sepsis (Croxen & Finlay, 2010). *P. aeruginosa* is involved in CF disease, which is already discussed in this chapter. *E. coli* and *P. aeruginosa* induce NOX-dependent suicidal NETosis by activating NADPH oxidase 2 (Nox), which subsequently generates ROS to induce NET (Khan, Philip, Cheung, Vadakepeedika, Grasemann, Sweezey, & Palaniyar, 2017).

Gastroenteritis is caused by *Salmonella typhimurium*, a Gram-negative bacterium known to stimulate NETosis (Brinkmann et al., 2004). Besides trapping and killing bacteria, active components of extracellular traps can neutralize virulence factors. *Mycobacterium tuberculosis*, an intracellular bacterium is capable of successfully evading the host immune system and to establish latent infection. While NETs trapped *M. tuberculosis*, the bacteria were not killed but there are some evidence that underlined the importance of neutrophils in containing the infection (Nandi & Behar, 2011) and suggest that NETs may be physically restricting *M. tuberculosis*. This hypothesis needs further investigation in animal models and human studies.

Fungal diseases

Neutrophils play a crucial role in containing fungal infections and NETs appear to be an important part of the neutrophil antifungal arsenal. *Candida albicans* causes disease in immunecompromised subjects, such as patients with pancreatitis or renal insufficiency, patients on antibiotic treatment or with a central venous catheter, and in patients following gastrointestinal surgery. Neutrophils can trap and eliminate *C. albicans* in either its yeast or hyphal form by releasing NETs (Mayer, Wilson, & Hube, 2013; Urban et al., 2006).

Cryptococcosis and meningoencephalitis caused by pathogenic yeast, *Cryptococcus neoformans*, possesses a capsular polysaccharide that confers it with the ability to regulate the host immune system and is able to modulate NET production.

Chronic granulomatous disease (CGD), an inherited disorder of NADPH oxidase, is characterized by recurrent life-threatening bacterial and fungal infections. It has the highest invasive aspergillosis infections by *A. fumigatus*, a part of human microbiota which stimulates NETs induction through NOX activation (Bianchi et al., 2009). CGD patients are deficient in the expression of NADPH oxidase and not able to form NET and die due to *Aspergillus nidulans* infection. Bianchi et al., 2009 have indicated that *A. nidulans* conidia can be killed by the help of NETs.

Parasitic diseases

Studies have reported the potential role of NETs in the immune response against protozoan parasites. Causing agent of malaria is *Plasmodium falciparum* that induces the production of inflammatory cytokines by infected erythrocytes. The invasion of the parasites is facilitated by proteins expressed on the infected erythrocytes which promote their adhesion to the vascular endothelium in tissues and organs. The presence of NETs and the formation of antinuclear antibodies may contribute to disease in the development of autoimmune phenotypes. The role of NETs has also been studied in parasites causing leishmaniasis. Leishmania parasites are the inducing agents in a variety of leishmaniasis infections where, depending on the species, the phenotype can range from cutaneous and subcutaneous lesions to potentially lethal visceral leishmaniasis (kala-azar). Depending on the species some Leishmaniasis parasites are killed by NET whereas some have developed strategies to evade the antimicrobial activity of

NET, for example, in humans, *Leishmania amazonensis* can induce NET formation and get killed by them, in contrast, *Leishmania infantum* and *Leishmania donovani* parasites do not get killed by NETs (Gabriel, McMaster, Girard, & Descoteaux, 2010).

NETosis is also implicated in *Toxoplasma gondii* infection, which occurs as a result of the ingestion of contaminated food. The parasitic infection stimulates neutrophils recruitment to the infected sites (Nathan et al., 2006) and induces NETs formation from human and mouse neutrophils. Entrapment of the parasite within NETs leads to the decreased parasite viability. NET formation checks *Toxoplasma* infection by direct microbicidal effects and by interfering with the parasite invasion of the target host cells.

Viral diseases

Several reports have examined that NETs have a role in viral infection such as human immunodeficiency virus 1 (HIV-1), dengue virus, influenza A virus, and respiratory syncytial virus. HIV-1 is a life-threatening virus that attacks the immune system. NET can capture and deactivate the negatively charged HIV virions and significantly decreased the activity of HIV infection. MPO and α-defensins are antiviral proteins associated with NET structures and may aid to entrap and eliminate HIV. HIV has an immune evasion mechanism, which promotes IL-10 production by DCs and thus preventing ROS production and NET formation (Saitoh et al., 2012).

In recent years, the incidence of dengue infection has increased worldwide. Dengue virus is a single-stranded RNA virus that has several dengue serotypes with effects that range from mild fever to severe dengue. It has been reported that dengue virus serotype-2 inhibits the formation of NET by the disruption of Glut-1—mediated glucose uptake (Moreno-Altamirano, Rodriguez-Espinosa, Rojas-Espinosa, PliegoRivero, & Sanchez-Garcia, 2015), a metabolic requirement for NET release (Rodriguez-Espinosa, Rojas-Espinosa, Moreno-Altamirano, LopezVillegas, & Sanchez-Garcia, 2015).

Pneumonia caused by *H. influenzae* is a deadly virus known for killing millions of people around the world. It is characterized by excessive neutrophils recruitment to the lungs, aided by CXCR2. It also stimulates PAD4-mediated NET formation (Hemmers, Teijaro, Arandjelovic, & Mowen, 2011). α-Defensin-1 associated with NETs inhibits virus replication by blocking PKC pathway.

Pediatric infection such as acute bronchitis, mucosal and submucosal edema, and luminal occlusion caused by a respiratory syncytial virus (RSV) (Borchers, Chang, Gershwin, & Gershwin, 2013). NET stimulated by this virus but unable to kill it (Cortjens et al., 2016). RSV F protein induces NET formation via the TLR4 pathway. Despite these NETs acting as viral reservoirs, their presence may aggravate inflammatory symptoms and promote luminal occlusion with structures composed of mucus and DNA (Funchal, Jaeger, Czepielewski, Machado, Muraro, & Stein, 2015).

In conclusion NETs are effective against a variety of microbes but may be critical against pathogens that are resistant against phagocytosis. It appears as a key mechanism in microbial trapping to prevent microbial dissemination. However, dysregulation of NET formation and clearance appears to have negative health effects.

In Vitro neutrophil extracellular trap formation: measurement techniques

In recent years various methods have emerged for evaluation of NET such as flow cytometry and histochemistry. NET flow cytometry method uses a plasma membrane−impermeable DNA-binding dye, SYTOX Green which can detect the green positive human peripheral polymorphonuclear cells exposed by NET inducer, phorbol 12-myristate 13-acetate (PMA). Diphenyleneiodonium is a NET inhibitor could significantly reduce the number of SYTOX Green−positive cells induced by PMA. Thus it suggested that SYTOX Green−positive cells include neutrophils that formed NET. This method could detect neutrophils that undergo NETosis, but it cannot be useful for early apoptosis.

For the evaluation of NET the most popular method is microscopic observation, a reliable method, which is based on the confirmation of colocalization of extracellular DNA and neutrophil-derived proteins, including MPO and NE, it has faults in objectivity and quantification. It is applicable for quantitative evaluation but subjective views on the results have to be avoided. Soluble NET remnants in fluid samples, such as serum and cell culture supernatants, have also been monitored for the quantity of NET. Cell-free DNA can be detected objectively and quantitatively using Picogreen (Zhang et al., 2014). Another technique is the enzyme-linked immunosorbent assay (ELISA) can detect the complexes of DNA and neutrophil-derived proteins, including MPO and NE, can be detected (Kessenbrock et al., 2009; Nakazawa et al., 2012). Moreover, sometimes soluble NET remnants do not reflect the NET formation in vivo accurately because degradation of NET by serum DNase I is disordered in some patients with SLE (Hakkim et al., 2010) and AAV (Nakazawa et al., 2014). Gavillet et al. (2015), recognized neutrophils that underwent NETosis by recognition of MPO and citrullinated histones utilizing flow cytometry. Zhao, Fogg, and Kaplan (2015), conducted multispectral imaging flow cytometry that can mainly detect the change of nuclear area and fluorescent intensity caused by NET. Although these are objective and quantitative methods, their protocols appear to be complex. For the study of NET, a simpler, objective, and quantitative method were used for detection of neutrophils that formed NET.

References

Abbott, N. J., Rönnbäck, L., & Hansson, E. (2006). Astrocyte-endothelial interactions at the blood-brain barrier. *Nature Review Neuroscience*, *7*(1), 41−53. Available from https://doi.org/10.1038/nrn1824.

Aghajanian, A., Wittchen, E. S., Campbell, S. L., & Burridge, K. (2009). Direct activation of RhoA by reactive oxygen species requires a redox-sensitive motif. *PLoS One*, *4*(11), e8045. Available from https://doi.org/10.1371/journal.pone.0008045.

Alexandraki, K. I., Piperi, C., Ziakas, P. D., Apostolopoulos, N. V., Makrilakis, K., Syriou, V., ... Kalofoutis, A. (2008). Cytokine secretion in long-standing diabetes mellitus type 1 and 2: associations with low-grade systemic inflammation. *Journal of Clinical Immunology*, *28*(4), 314−321. Available from https://doi.org/10.1007/s10875-007-9164-1.

Allen, C., Thornton, P., Denes, A., McColl, B. W., Pierozynski, A., Monestier, M., ... Allan, S. M. (2012). Neutrophil cerebrovascular transmigration triggers rapid neurotoxicity through release of proteases associated with decondensed DNA. *Journal of Immunology*, *189*(1), 381−392. Available from https://doi.org/10.4049/jimmunol.1200409.

Ammollo, C. T., Semeraro, F., Xu, J., Esmon, N. L., & Esmon, C. T. (2011). Extracellular histones increase plasma thrombin generation by impairing thrombomodulin-dependent protein C activation. *Journal of Thrombosis and Haemostasis*, *9*(9), 1795−1803. Available from https://doi.org/10.1111/j.1538-7836.2011.

Banks, P. A., Bollen, T. L., Dervenis, C., Gooszen, H. G., Johnson, C. D., Sarr, M. G., ... Acute Pancreatitis Classification Working Group. (2013). Classification of acute pancreatitis (2012): revision of the Atlanta classification and definitions by international consensus. *Gut*, *62*(1), 102−111. Available from https://doi.org/10.1136/gutjnl-2012-302779.

Bass, J. I. F., Russo, D. M., Gabelloni, M. L., Geffner, J. R., Giordano, M., & Catalano, M. (2010). Extracellular DNA: a major proinflammatory component of Pseudomonas aeruginosa biofilms. *Journal of Immunology*, *184*, 6386−6395. Available from https://doi.org/10.4049/jimmunol.0901640.

Beiter, K., Wartha, F., Albiger, B., Normark, S., Zychlinsky, A., & Henriques-Normark, B. (2006). An endonuclease allows Streptococcus pneumoniae to escape from neutrophil extracellular traps. *Current Biology*, *16*, 401−407. Available from https://doi.org/10.1016/j.cub.2006.01.056.

Berends, E. T., Horswill, A. R., Haste, N. M., Monestier, M., Nizet, V., & von Köckritz-Blickwede, M. (2010). Nuclease expression by *Staphylococcus aureus* facilitates escape from neutrophil extracellular traps. *Journal of Innate Immunology*, *2*(6), 576−586. Available from https://doi.org/10.1159/000319909.

Berezin, A. E. (2016a). Impaired immune phenotype of endothelial cell-derived microparticles: The missed link between diabetes-related states and risk of cardiovascular complications. *Journal of Data Mining in Genomics & Proteomics*, *7*, 195. Available from https://doi.org/10.4172/2153-0602.1000195.

Berezin, A. E. (2016b). Is the neutrophil extracellular trap-driven microvascular inflammation essential for diabetes vasculopathy. *Biomedical Research and Therapy*, *3*(5), 618−624.

Berezin, A. E. (2016c). The neutrophil extracellular traps: The missed link between microvascular inflammation and diabetes. *Metabolomics*, *6*(1), 1−3. Available from https://doi.org/10.4172/2153-0769.1000163.

Berger-Achituv, S., Brinkmann, V., Abed, U. A., Kühn, L. I., Ben-Ezra, J., Elhasid, R., & Zychlinsky, A. (2013). A proposed role for neutrophil extracellular traps in cancer immunoediting. *Frontiers in Immunology*, *4*, 48. Available from https://doi.org/10.3389/fimmu.2013.00048.

Bianchi, M., Hakkim, A., Brinkmann, V., Siler, U., Seger, R. A., Zychlinsky, A., & Reichenbach, J. (2009). Restoration of NET formation by gene therapy in CGD controls aspergillosis. *Blood*, *114*(13), 2619−2622. Available from https://doi.org/10.1182/blood-2009-05-221606.

Bianchi, M., Niemiec, M. J., Siler, U., Urban, C. F., & Reichenbach, J. (2011). Restoration of anti-*Aspergillus* defense by neutrophil extracellular traps in human chronic granulomatous disease after gene therapy is calprotectin-dependent. *Journal of Allergy and Clinical Immunology*, *127*(5), 1243−1252.

Borchers, A. T., Chang, C., Gershwin, M. E., & Gershwin, L. J. (2013). Respiratory syncytial virus − a comprehensive review. *Clinical Reviews in Allergy Immunology*, *45*, 331−379. Available from https://doi.org/10.1007/s12016-013-8368-9

Brandt, T., Breitenstein, S., von der Hardt, H., & Tummler, B. (1995). DNA concentration and length in sputum of patients with cystic fibrosis during inhalation with recombinant human DNase. *Thorax*, *50*(8), 880−882. Available from https://doi.org/10.1136/thx.50.8.880.

Branzk, N., Lubojemska, A., Hardison, S. E., Wang, Q., Gutierrez, M. G., Brown, G. D., & Papayannopoulos, V. (2014). Neutrophils sense microbe size and selectively release neutrophil extracellular traps in response to large pathogens. *Nature Immunology*, *15*(11), 1017−1025.

Brinkmann, V., Reichard, U., Goosmann, C., Fauler, B., Uhlemann, Y., Weiss, D. S., ... Zychlinsky, A. (2004). Neutrophil extracellular traps kill bacteria. *Science*, *303*(5663), 1532−1535. Available from https://doi.org/10.1126/science.1092385.

Bruns, S., Kniemeyer, O., Hasenberg, M., Aimanianda, V., Nietzsche, S., Tywissen, A., ... Gunzer, M. (2010). Production of extracellular traps against *Aspergillus fumigatus* in vitro and in infected lung tissue is dependent on invading neutrophils and influenced by hydrophobin RodA. *PLOS Pathogens*, *6*(4), e1000873. Available from https://doi.org/10.1371/journal.ppat.1000873.

Buter, A., Imrie, C. W., Carter, C. R., Evans, S., & McKay, C. J. (2002). Dynamic nature of early organ dysfunction determines outcome in acute pancreatitis. *British Journal of Surger*, *89*(3), 298−302. Available from https://doi.org/10.1046/j.0007-1323.2001.

Caprnda, M., Mesarosova, D., Ortega, P. F., Krahulec, B., Egom, E., Rodrigo, L., ... Gaspar, L. (2017). Glycemic variability and vascular complications in patients with type 2 diabetes mellitus. *Folia Medica*, *59*(3), 270−278.

Carestia, A., Frechtel, G., Cerrone, G., Linari, M. A., Gonzalez, C. D., Casais, P., & Schattner, M. (2016). NETosis before and after hyperglycemic control in type 2 diabetes mellitus patients. *PLoS One*, *11*(12), e0168647.

Chatfield, S. M., Grebe, K., Whitehead, L. W., Rogers, K. L., Nebl, T., Murphy, J. M., & Wicks, I. P. (2018). Monosodium urate crystals generate nuclease-resistant neutrophil extracellular traps via a distinct molecular pathway. *Journal of Immunology*, *200*(5), 1802−1816. Available from https://doi.org/10.4049/jimmunol.1701382.

Chaurio, R. A., Munoz, L. E., Maueroder, C., Janko, C., Harrer, T., Furnrohr, B. G., ... Berens, C. (2014). The progression of cell death affects the rejection of allogeneic tumors in immune-competent mice—implications for cancer therapy. *Frontiers in Immunology*, *5*, 560. Available from https://doi.org/10.3389/fmmu.2014.00560.

Clark, S. R., Ma, A. C., Tavener, S. A., McDonald, B., Goodarzi, Z., Kelly, M. M., ... Kubes, P. (2007). Platelet TLR4 activates neutrophil extracellular traps to ensnare bacteria in septic blood. *Nature Medicine*, *13*(4), 463−469. Available from https://doi.org/10.1038/nm1565.

Cools-Lartigue, J., Spicer, J., McDonald, B., Gowing, S., Chow, S., Giannias, B., ... Ferri, L. (2013). Neutrophil extracellular traps sequester circulating tumor cells and promote metastasis. *Journal of Clinical Investigation*, *123*, 3446−3458. Available from https://doi.org/10.1172/JCI67484.

Cortjens, B., de Boer, O. J., de Jong, R., Antonis, A. F., Sabogal Piñeros, Y. S., Lutter, R., ... Bem, R. A. (2016). Neutrophil extracellular traps cause airway obstruction during respiratory syncytial virus disease. *The Journal of Pathology, 238*(3), 401−411. Available from https://doi.org/10.1002/path.4660.

Cronstein, B. N., & Sunkureddi, P. (2013). Mechanistic aspects of inflammation and clinical management of inflammation in acute gouty arthritis. *Journal of Clinical Rheumatology, 19*(1), 19−29.

Croxen, M. A., & Finlay, B. B. (2010). Molecular mechanisms of Escherichia coli pathogenicity. *Nature Reviews Microbiology, 8*, 26−38. Available from https://doi.org/10.1038/nrmicro2265.

Czirr, E., & Wyss-Coray, T. (2012). The immunology of neurodegeneration. *Journal of Clinical Investigation, 122*(4), 1156−1163. Available from https://doi.org/10.1172/JCI58656.

de Boer, O. J., Li, X., Teeling, P., Mackaay, C., Ploegmakers, H. J., van der Loos, C. M., ... van der Wal, A. C. (2013). Neutrophils, neutrophil extracellular traps and interleukin-17 associate with the organisation of thrombi in acute myocardial infarction. *Thrombosis and Haemostasis, 109*(2), 290−297. Available from https://doi.org/10.1160/TH12-06-0425.

Delgado-Rizo, V., Martínez-Guzmán, M. A., Iñiguez-Gutierrez, L., García-Orozco, A., Alvarado-Navarro, A., & Fafutis-Morris, M. (2017). Neutrophil extracellular traps and its implications in inflammation: An overview. *Frontiers in Immunology, 8*, 81. Available from https://doi.org/10.3389/fimmu.2017.00081.

Demers, M., Krause, D. S., Schatzberg, D., Martinod, K., Voorhees, J. R., Fuchs, T. A., ... Wagner, D. D. (2012). Cancers predispose neutrophils to release extracellular DNA traps that contribute to cancer-associated thrombosis. *PNAS, 109*(32), 13076−13081. Available from https://doi.org/10.1073/pnas.1200419109.

Demers, M., & Wagner, D. D. (2013). Neutrophil extracellular traps: A new link to cancer-associated thrombosis and potential implications for tumor progression. *OncoImmunology, 2*(2), e22946.

Desai, J., Foresto-Neto, O., Honarpisheh, M., Steiger, S., Nakazawa, D., Popper, B., ... Anders, H. J. (2017). Particles of different sizes and shapes induce neutrophil necroptosis followed by the release of neutrophil extracellular trap-like chromatin. *Scientific Reports, 7*(1), 15003. Available from https://doi.org/10.1038/s41598-017-15106-0.

Desai, J., Mulay, S. R., Nakazawa, D., & Anders, H. J. (2016). Matters of life and death. How neutrophils die or survive along NET release and is "NETosis" = necroptosis? *Cellular and Molecular Life Sciences, 73*(11−12), 2211−2219.

Dubois, A. V., Gauthier, A., Brea, D., Varaigne, F., Diot, P., Gauthier, F., & Attucci, S. (2012). Influence of DNA on the activities and inhibition of neutrophil serine proteases in cystic fibrosis sputum. *American Journal of Respiratory Cell and Molecular Biology, 47*(1), 80−86. Available from https://doi.org/10.1165/rcmb.2011-0380OC.

Dwyer, M., Shan, Q., D'Ortona, S., Maurer, R., Mitchell, R., Olesen, H., ... Gadjeva, M. (2014). Cystic fibrosis sputum DNA has NETosis characteristics and neutrophil extracellular trap release is regulated by macrophage migration-inhibitory factor. *Journal of Innate Immunology, 6*(6), 765−779. Available from https://doi.org/10.1159/000363242.

Fadini, G. P., Menegazzo, L., Rigato, M., Scattolini, V., Poncina, N., Bruttocao, A., ... Avogaro, A. (2016). NETosis delays diabetic wound healing in mice and humans. *Diabetes, 65*(4), 1061−1071. Available from https://doi.org/10.2337/db15-0863.

Fadini, G. P., Menegazzo, L., Scattolini, V., Gintoli, M., Albiero, M., & Avogaro, A. (2016). A perspective on NETosis in diabetes and cardiometabolic disorders. *Nutrition, Metabolism & Cardiovascular Diseases, 26*(1), 1−8.

Forlenza, O. V., Diniz, B. S., Talib, L. L., Mendonça, V. A., Ojopi, E. B., Gattaz, W. F., & Teixeira, A. L. (2009). Increased serum IL-1beta level in Alzheimer's disease and mild cognitive impairment. *Dementia and Geriatric Cognitive Disorders*, *28*(6), 507−512. Available from https://doi.org/10.1159/000255051.

Freigang, S., Ampenberger, F., Weiss, A., Kanneganti, T. D., Iwakura, Y., Hersberger, M., & Kopf, M. (2013). Fatty acid-induced mitochondrial uncoupling elicits inflammasome independent IL-1a and sterile vascular inflammation in atherosclerosis. *Nature Immunology*, *14* (10), 1045−1053.

Funchal, G. A., Jaeger, N., Czepielewski, R. S., Machado, M. S., Muraro, S. P., & Stein, R. T. (2015). Respiratory syncytial virus fusion protein promotes TLR-4-dependent neutrophil extracellular trap formation by human neutrophils. *PLoS One*, *10*. Available from https://doi.org/10.1371/journal.pone.0124082, e0124082.

Fuchs, H. J., Borowitz, D. S., Christiansen, D. H., Morris, E. M., Nash, M. L., Ramsey, B. W., . . . Wohl, M. E. (1994). Effect of aerosolized recombinant human DNase on exacerbations of respiratory symptoms and on pulmonary function in patients with cystic fibrosis. *The New England Journal of Medicine*, *331*(10), 637−642.

Fuchs, T. A., Abed, U., Goosmann, C., Hurwitz, R., Schulze, I., Wahn, V., . . . Zychlinsky, A. (2007). Novel cell death program leads to neutrophil extracellular traps. *The Journal of Cell Biology*, *176*(2), 231−241.

Fuchs, T. A., Brill, A., Duerschmied, D., Schatzberg, D., Monestier, M., Myers, D. D., Jr., . . . Wagner, D. D. (2010). Extracellular DNA traps promote thrombosis. *PNAS*, *107*(36), 15880−15885. Available from https://doi.org/10.1073/pnas.1005743107.

Gabriel, C., McMaster, W. R., Girard, D., & Descoteaux, A. (2010). *Leishmania donovani* promastigotes evade the antimicrobial activity of neutrophil extracellular traps. *Journal of Immunology*, *185*(7), 4319−4327. Available from https://doi.org/10.4049/jimmunol.1000893.

Garg, A. D., Galluzzi, L., Apetoh, L., Baert, T., Birge, R. B., Bravo-San Pedro, J. M., . . . Agostinis, P. (2015). Molecular and translational classifications of DAMPs in immunogenic cell death. *Frontiers in Immunology*, *6*, 588. Available from https://doi.org/10.3389/fimmu.2015.00588.

Gavillet, M., Martinod, K., Renella, R., Harris, C., Shapiro, N. I., Wagner, D. D., & Williams, D. A. (2015). Flow cytometric assay for direct quantification of neutrophil extracellular traps in blood samples. *American Journal of Hematology*, *90*(12), 1155−1158. Available from https://doi.org/10.1002/ajh.24185.

Gazendam, R. P., van Hamme, J. L., Tool, A. T., Hoogenboezem, M., van den Berg, J. M., Prins, J. M., . . . Kuijpers, T. W. (2016). Human neutrophils use different mechanisms to kill *Aspergillus fumigatus* conidia and hyphae: evidence from phagocyte defects. *Journal of Immunology*, *196*(3), 1272−1283. Available from https://doi.org/10.4049/jimmunol.1501811.

Giri, R., Shen, Y., Stins, M., Du Yan, S., Schmidt, A. M., Stern, D., . . . Kalra, V. K. (2000). Beta-amyloid-induced migration of monocytes across human brain endothelial cells involves RAGE and PECAM-1. *American Journal of Physiology-Cell Physiology*, *279*(6), C1772−C1781.

Gonzalez, D. J., Corriden, R., Akong-Moore, K., Olson, J., Dorrestein, P. C., & Nizet, V. (2014). N-terminal ArgD peptides from the classical Staphylococcus aureus agr system have cytotoxic and proinflammatory activities. *Chemical Biology*, *21*, 1457−1462. Available from https://doi.org/10.1016/j.chembiol.2014.09.015.

Gould, T. J., Vu, T. T., Swystun, L. L., Dwivedi, D. J., Mai, S. H., Weitz, J. I., & Liaw, P. C. (2014). Neutrophil extracellular traps promote thrombin generation through platelet-dependent and platelet-independent mechanisms. *Arteriosclerosis', Thrombosis, and Vascular Biology*, *34*(9), 1977−1984. Available from https://doi.org/10.1161/ATVBAHA.114.304114.

Grammas, P., & Ovase, R. (2001). Inflammatory factors are elevated in brain microvessels in Alzheimer's disease. *Neurobiology of Aging*, *22*(6), 837−842. Available from https://doi.org/10.1016/S0197-4580(01)00276-7.

Grammas, P., Samany, P. G., & Tirumangalakudi, L. (2006). Thrombin and inflammatory proteins are elevated in Alzheimer's disease microvessels: Implications for disease pathogenesis. *Journal of Alzheimer's Disease*, *9*(1), 51−58.

Gray, R. D., McCullagh, B. N., & McCray, P. B. (2015). NETs and CF lung disease: Current status and future prospects. *Antibiotics (Basel)*, *4*(1), 62−75. Available from https://doi.org/10.3390/antibiotics4010062.

Gregory, A. D., & Houghton, A. M. (2011). Tumor-associated neutrophils: new targets for cancer therapy. *Cancer Research*, *71*(7), 2411−2416. Available from https://doi.org/10.1158/0008-5472.

Griffin, W. S., Stanley, L. C., Ling, C., White, L., MacLeod, V., Perrot, L. J., ... Araoz, C. (1989). Brain interleukin 1 and S-100 immunoreactivity are elevated in Down syndrome and Alzheimer disease. *PNAS*, *86*(19), 7611−7615. Available from https://doi.org/10.1073/pnas.86.19.7611.

Hakkim, A., Furnrohr, B. G., Amann, K., Laube, B., Abed, U. A., Brinkmann, V., ... Zychlinsky, A. (2010). Impairment of neutrophil extracellular trap degradation is associated with lupus nephritis. *PNAS*, *107*(21), 9813−9818. Available from https://doi.org/10.1073/pnas.0909927107.

Halonen, K. I., Pettila, V., Leppaniemi, A. K., Kemppainen, E. A., Puolakkainen, P. A., & Haapiainen, R. K. (2002). Multiple organ dysfunction associated with severe acute pancreatitis. *Critical Care Medicine*, *30*(6), 1274−1279. Available from https://doi.org/10.1097/00003246-200206000-00019.

Hanses, F., Park, S., Rich, J., & Lee, J. C. (2011). Reduced neutrophil apoptosis in diabetic mice during staphylococcal infection leads to prolonged TNFα production and reduced neutrophil clearance. *PLoS One*, *6*, e23633. Available from https://doi.org/10.1371/journal.pone.0023633.

Hemmers, S., Teijaro, J. R., Arandjelovic, S., & Mowen, K. A. (2011). PAD4-mediated neutrophil extracellular trap formation is not required for immunity against influenza infection. *PLoS One*, *6*, e22043. Available from https://doi.org/10.1371/journal.pone.0022043.

Heneka, M. T., Carson, M. J., El Khoury, J., Landreth, G. E., Brosseron, F., Feinstein, D. L., ... Kummer, M. P. (2015). Neuroinflammation in Alzheimer's disease. *The Lancet Neurology*, *14*(4), 388−405. Available from https://doi.org/10.1016/S1474-4422(15)70016-5.

Heppner, F. L., Ransohoff, R. M., & Becher, B. (2015). Immune attack: the role of inflammation in Alzheimer disease. *Nature Review Neuroscience*, *16*(6), 358−372. Available from https://doi.org/10.1038/nrn3880.

Herrick, S., Ashcroft, G., Ireland, G., Horan, M., McCollum, C., & Ferguson, M. (1997). Upregulation of elastase in acute wounds of healthy aged humans and chronic venous leg ulcers are associated with matrix degradation. *Laboratory Investigation*, *77*(3), 281−288.

Holmin, S., Söderlund, J., Biberfeld, P., & Mathiesen, T. (1998). Intracerebral inflammation after human brain contusion. *Neurosurgery*, *42*(2), 291−298, discussion 298−9.

Hubbard, R. C., McElvaney, N. G., Birrer, P., Shak, S., Robinson, W. W., Jolley, C., ... Crystal, R. G. (1992). A preliminary study of aerosolized recombinant human deoxyribonuclease I in the treatment of cystic fibrosis. *The New England Journal of Medicine*, *326*(12), 812−815.

Itoh, Y., & Nagase, H. (1995). Preferential inactivation of tissue inhibitor of metalloproteinases-1 that is bound to the precursor of matrix metalloproteinase 9 (progelatinase B) by human neutrophil elastase. *The Journal of Biological Chemistry*, *270*(28), 16518−16521. Available from https://doi.org/10.1074/jbc.270.28.16518.

Jenne, C. N., Urrutia, R., & Kubes, P. (2013). Platelets: Bridging hemostasis, inflammation, and immunity. *International Journal of Laboratory Hematology*, *35*(3), 254−261. Available from https://doi.org/10.1111/ijlh.12084.

Johnson, C. D., & Abu-Hilal, M. (2004). Persistent organ failure during the first week as a marker of fatal outcome in acute pancreatitis. *Gut*, *53*(9), 1340−1344. Available from https://doi.org/10.1136/gut.2004.039883.

Johnson, C. D., Kingsnorth, A. N., Imrie, C. W., McMahon, M. J., Neoptolemos, J. P., McKay, C., . . . Curtis, L. D. (2001). Double blind, randomised, placebo controlled study of a platelet activating factor antagonist, lexipafant, in the treatment and prevention of organ failure in predicted severe acute pancreatitis. *Gut.*, *48*(1), 62−69. Available from https://doi.org/10.1136/gut.48.1.62.

Joshi, M. B., Baipadithaya, G., Balakrishnan, A., Hegde, M., Vohra, M., Ahamed, R., . . . Satyamoorthy, K. (2016). Elevated homocysteine levels in type 2 diabetes induce constitutive neutrophil extracellular traps. *Scientific Reports*, *6*, 36362. Available from https://doi.org/10.1038/srep36362.

Kakuta, K., Dohi, K., Miyoshi, M., Yamanaka, T., Kawamura, M., Masuda, J., . . . Ito, M. (2017). Impact of renal function on the underlying pathophysiology of coronary plaque composition in patients with type 2 diabetes mellitus. *Cardiovascular Diabetology*, *16*(1), 131. Available from https://doi.org/10.1186/s12933-017-0618-3.

Kambas, K., Chrysanthopoulou, A., Vassilopoulos, D., Apostolidou, E., Skendros, P., Girod, A., . . . Ritis, K. (2013). Tissue factor expression in neutrophil extracellular traps and neutrophil derived microparticles in antineutrophil cytoplasmic antibody associated vasculitis may promote thromboinflammation and the thrombophilic state associated with the disease. *Annals of the Rheumatic Diseases*, *73*(10), 1854−1863. Available from https://doi.org/10.1136/annrheumdis-2013-203430.

Kambas, K., Mitroulis, I., Apostolidou, E., Girod, A., Chrysanthopoulou, A., Pneumatikos, I., . . . Ritis, K. (2012). Autophagy mediates the delivery of thrombogenic tissue factor to neutrophil extracellular traps in human sepsis. *PLoS One*, *7*(9), e45427. Available from https://doi.org/10.1371/journal.pone.0045427.

Karima, M., Kantarci, A., Ohira, T., Hasturk, H., Jones, V. L., Nam, B. H., . . . Van Dyke, T. E. (2005). Enhanced superoxide release and elevated protein kinase C activity in neutrophils from diabetic patients: Association with periodontitis. *Journal of Leukocyte Biology*, *78*(4), 862−870.

Keenan, R. T., O'Brien, W. R., Lee, K. H., Crittenden, D. B., Fisher, M. C., Goldfarb, D. S., . . . Pillinger, M. H. (2011). Prevalence of contraindications and prescription of pharmacologic therapies for gout. *The American Journal of Medicine*, *124*(2), 155−163.

Kelly, K. A., Setlur, S. R., Ross, R., Anbazhagan, R., Waterman, P., Rubin, M. A., & Weissleder, R. (2008). Detection of early prostate cancer using a hepsin-targeted imaging agent. *Cancer Research*, *68*(7), 2286−2291.

Kenne, E., Erlandsson, A., Lindbom, L., Hillered, L., & Clausen, F. (2012). Neutrophil depletion reduces edema formation and tissue loss following traumatic brain injury in mice. *Journal of Neuroinflammation*, *9*, 17. Available from https://doi.org/10.1186/1742-2094-9-17.

Kenny, E. F., Herzig, A., Krüger, R., Muth, A., Mondal, S., Thompson, P. R., . . . Zychlinsky, A. (2017). Diverse stimuli engage different neutrophil extracellular trap pathways. *Elife*, *6*, e24437. Available from https://doi.org/10.7554/eLife.24437.

Keshari, R. S., Jyoti, A., Dubey, M., Kothari, N., Kohli, M., Bogra, J., . . . Dikshit, M. (2012). Cytokines induced neutrophil extracellular traps formation: implication for the inflammatory disease condition. *PLoS One*, *7*(10), 1−8. Available from https://doi.org/10.1371/journal.pone.0048111.

Kessenbrock, K., Krumbholz, M., Schonermarck, U., Back, W., Gross, W. L., Werb, Z., . . . Jenne, D. E. (2009). Netting neutrophils in autoimmune small-vessel vasculitis. *Nature Medicine.*, *15*(6), 623−625. Available from https://doi.org/10.1038/nm.1959.

Khan, M. A., Philip, L. M., Cheung, G., Vadakepeedika, S., Grasemann, H., Sweezey, N., & Palaniyar, N. (2018). Regulating NETosis: Increasing pH Promotes NADPH Oxidase-Dependent NETosis. *Frontiers in Medicine*, *5*, 19. Available from https://doi.org/10.3389/fmed.2018.00019.

Khandpur, R., Carmona-Rivera, C., Vivekanandan-Giri, A., Gizinski, A., Yalavarthi, S., Knight, J. S., . . . Kaplan, M. J. (2013). NETs are a source of citrullinated autoantigens and stimulate inflammatory responses in rheumatoid arthritis. *Science Translation Medicine*, *5*(178). Available from https://doi.org/10.1126/scitranslmed.3005580, pp. 178ra40.

Khanna, D., Fitzgerald, J. D., Khanna, P. P., Bae, S., Singh, M. K., Neogi, T., . . . American College of Rheumatology. (2012). 2012 American College of Rheumatology guidelines for management of gout. Part 1: Systematic nonpharmacologic and pharmacologic therapeutic approaches to hyperuricemia. *Arthritis Care & Research*, *64*(10), 1431−1446.

Klebanoff, S. J., Kinsella, M. G., & Wight, T. N. (1993). Degradation of endothelial cell matrix heparan sulfate proteoglycan by elastase and the myeloperoxidase-H_2O_2-chloride system. *The American Journal of Pathology*, *143*(3), 907−917.

Konstan, M. W., & Ratjen, F. (2012). Effect of dornase alfa on inflammation and lung function: potential role in the early treatment of cystic fibrosis. *Journal of Cystic Fibrosis*, *11*(2), 78−83.

Konstan, M. W., Wagener, J. S., Pasta, D. J., Millar, S. J., Jacobs, J. R., Yegin, A., . . . Scientific advisory group and investigators and coordinators of epidemiologic study of cystic fibrosis. (2011). Clinical use of dornase alpha is associated with a slower rate of FEV1 decline in cystic fibrosis. *Pediatric Pulmonology*, *46*(6), 545−553. Available from https://doi.org/10.1002/ppul.21388.

Kumar, V., & Sharma, A. (2010). Neutrophils: Cinderella of innate immune system. *International Immunopharmacology*, *10*(11), 1325−1334. Available from https://doi.org/10.1016/j.intimp.2010.08.012.

Kylanpaa, M. L., Mentula, P., Kemppainen, E., Puolakkainen, P., Aittomaki, S., Silvennoinen, O., . . . Repo, H. (2005). Monocyte anergy is present in patients with severe acute pancreatitis and is significantly alleviated by granulocyte-macrophage colony-stimulating factor and interferon-gamma in vitro. *Pancreas*, *31*(1), 23−27. Available from https://doi.org/10.1097/01.mpa.0000164449.23524.94.

Law, S. M., & Gray, R. D. (2017). Neutrophil extracellular traps and the dysfunctional innate immune response of cystic fibrosis lung disease: a review. *Journal of Inflammation*, *14*, 29. Available from https://doi.org/10.1186/s12950-017-0176-1.

Leavy, O. (2015). Inflammation: NETing a one-two punch. *Nature Reviews Immunology*, *15*(9), 526−527.

Lehoux, S., & Jones, E. A. (2016). Shear stress, arterial identity and atherosclerosis. *Thrombosis and Haemostasis*, *115*(3), 467−473. Available from https://doi.org/10.1160/TH15-10-0791.

Lieberman, J. (1968). Dornase aerosol effect on sputum viscosity in cases of cystic fibrosis. *JAMA*, *205*(5), 312−313.

Lip, G. Y., Chin, B. S., & Blann, A. D. (2002). Cancer and the prothrombotic state. *The Lancet Oncology*, *3*(1), 27−34. Available from https://doi.org/10.1016/S1470-2045(01)00619-2.

Liu, G. Y. (2009). Molecular pathogenesis of Staphylococcus aureus infection. *Pediatric Research*, *65*, 71R−77RR. Available from https://doi.org/10.1203/PDR.0b013e31819dc44d.

Longstaff, C., Varju, I., Sotonyi, P., Szabom, L., Krumrey, M., Hoell, A., . . . Kolev, K. (2013). Mechanical stability and fibrinolytic resistance of clots containing fibrin, DNA, and histones. *The Journal of Biological Chemistry*, *288*(10), 6946–6956. Available from https://doi.org/10.1074/jbc.M112.404301.

Love, S. (2010). Contribution of cerebral amyloid angiopathy to Alzheimer's disease. *Journal of Neurology, Neurosurgery, and Psychiatry*, *75*(1), 1–4.

Maksimow, M., Kyhala, L., Nieminen, A., Kylänpää, L., Aalto, K., Elima, K., ... Salmi, M. (2014). Early prediction of persistent organ failure by soluble CD73 in patients with acute pancreatitis*. *Critical Care Medicine*, *42*(12), 2556–2564. Available from https://doi.org/10.1097/CCM.0000000000000550.

Malachowa, N., Kobayashi, S. D., Freedman, B., Dorward, D. W., & DeLeo, F. R. (2013). Staphylococcus aureus leukotoxin GH promotes formation of neutrophil extracellular traps. *Journal of Immunology*, *191*, 6022–6029.

Mangold, A., Alias, S., Scherz, T., Hofbauer, T., Jakowitsch, J., Panzenbock, A., ... Lang, I. M. (2015). Coronary neutrophil extracellular trap burden and deoxyribonuclease activity in ST-elevation acute coronary syndrome are predictors of ST-segment resolution and infarct size. *Circulation Research*, *116*(7), 1182–1192.

Manzenreiter, R., Kienberger, F., Marcos, V., Schilcher, K., Krautgartner, W. D., Obermayer, A., ... Hartl, D. (2012). Ultrastructural characterization of cystic fibrosis sputum using atomic force and scanning electron microscopy. *Journal of Cystic Fibrosis*, *11*(2), 84–92. Available from https://doi.org/10.1016/j.jcf.2011.09.008.

Marcos, V., Zhou-Suckow, Z., Önder Yildirim, A., Bohla, A., Hector, A., Vitkov, L., ... Hartl, D. (2015). Free DNA in cystic fibrosis airway fluids correlates with airflow obstruction. *Mediators of Inflammation*, *2015*, 408935. Available from https://doi.org/10.1155/2015/408935.

Martínez-Alemán, S. R., Campos-García, L., Palma-Nicolas, J. P., Hernández-Bello, R., González, G. M., & Sánchez-González, A. (2017). Understanding the entanglement: Neutrophil extracellular traps (NETs) in cystic fibrosis. *Frontiers in Cellular and Infection Microbiology*, *7*, 104. Available from https://doi.org/10.3389/fcimb.2017.00104.

Martinon, F., Petrilli, V., Mayor, A., Tardivel, A., & Tschopp, J. (2006). Gout-associated uric acid crystals activate the NALP3 inflammasome. *Nature*, *440*(7081), 237–241.

Mayer, F. L., Wilson, D., & Hube, B. (2013). Candida albicans pathogenicity mechanisms. *Virulence*, *4*(2), 119–128. Available from https://doi.org/10.4161/viru.22913.

McKay, C. J., & Buter, A. (2003). Natural history of organ failure in acute pancreatitis. *Pancreatology*, *3*(2), 111–114. Available from https://doi.org/10.1159/000070078.

Medical Advisory Secretariat. (2010). Stenting for peripheral artery disease of the lower extremities: An evidence-based analysis. *Ontario Health Technology Assessment Series*, *10*(18), 1–88.

Megens, R. T., Vijayan, S., Lievens, D., Doring, Y., van Zandvoort, M. A., Grommes, J., ... Soehnlein, O. (2012). Presence of luminal neutrophil extracellular traps in atherosclerosis. *Thrombosis and Haemostasis*, *107*(3), 597–598.

Menegazzo, L., Ciciliot, S., Poncina, N., Mazzucato, M., Persano, M., Bonora, B., ... Fadini, G. P. (2015). NETosis is induced by high glucose and associated with type 2 diabetes. *Acta Diabetologica*, *52*(3), 497–503. Available from https://doi.org/10.1007/s00592-014-0676-x.

Merza, M., Hartman, H., Rahman, M., Hwaiz, R., Zhang, E., Renström, E., ... Thorlacius, H. (2015). Neutrophil extracellular traps induce trypsin activation, inflammation, and tissue damage in mice with severe acute pancreatitis. *Gastroenterology*, *149*(7), 1920–1931. Available from https://doi.org/10.1053/j.gastro.2015.08.026.

Miller, N. M., Wang, J., Tan, Y., & Dittel, B. N. (2015). Anti-inflammatory mechanisms of IFN-γ studied in experimental autoimmune encephalomyelitis reveal neutrophils as a potential target in multiple sclerosis. *Frontiers in Neuroscience*, *9*, 287. Available from https://doi.org/10.3389/fnins.2015.00287.

Misawa, T., Takahama, M., Kozaki, T., Takayama, M., Kozaki, T., Lee, H., ... Akira, S. (2013). Microtubule-driven spatial arrangement of mitochondria promotes activation of the NLRP3 inflammasome. *Nature Immunology, 14*(5), 454–460.

Mitroulis, I., Kambas, K., Chrysanthopoulou, A., Skendros, P., Apostolidou, E., Kourtzelis, I., ... Konstantinos, R. (2011). Neutrophil extracellular trap formation is associated with IL-1β and autophagy-related signaling in gout. *PLoS One, 6*(12), e29318. Available from https://doi.org/10.1371/journal.pone.0029318.

Mitton-Fitzgerald, E., Gohr, C. M., Bettendorf, B., & Rosenthal, A. K. (2016). The role of ANK in calcium pyrophosphate deposition disease. *Current Rheumatology Report, 18*(5), 25. Available from https://doi.org/10.1007/s11926-016-0574-z.

Mohammedi, K., Woodward, M., Hirakawa, Y., Zoungas, S., Colagiuri, S., Hamet, P., ... Advance Collaborative Group. (2016). Presentations of major peripheral arterial disease and risk of major outcomes in patients with type 2 diabetes: Results from the ADVANCE-ON study. *Cardiovascular Diabetology, 15*(1), 129. Available from https://doi.org/10.1186/s12933-016-0446-x.

Moorthy, A. N., Narasaraju, T., Rai, P., Perumalsamy, R., Tan, K. B., & Wang, S. (2013). In vivo and in vitro studies on the roles of neutrophil extracellular traps during secondary pneumococcal pneumonia after primary pulmonary influenza infection. *Frontiers in Immunology, 4*, 56. Available from https://doi.org/10.3389/fmmu.2013.00056.

Moorthy, A. N., Rai, P., Jiao, H., Wang, S., Tan, K. B., & Qin, L. (2016). Capsules of virulent pneumococcal serotypes enhance formation of neutrophil extracellular traps during in vivo pathogenesis of pneumonia. *Oncotarget, 7*, 19327–19340. Available from https://doi.org/10.18632/oncotarget.8451.

Moreno-Altamirano, M. M., Rodriguez-Espinosa, O., Rojas-Espinosa, O., PliegoRivero, B., & Sanchez-Garcia, F. J. (2015). Dengue virus serotype-2 interferes with the formation of neutrophil extracellular traps. *Intervirology, 58*, 250–259. Available from https://doi.org/10.1159/000440723.

Mulay, S. R., Desai, J., Kumar, S. V., Eberhard, J. N., Thomasova, D., Romoli, S., ... Anders, H. J. (2016). Cytotoxicity of crystals involves RIPK3-MLKL-mediated necroptosis. *Nature Communication, 7*, 10274. Available from https://doi.org/10.1038/ncomms10274.

Nachat, R., Méchin, M. C., Takahara, H., Chavanas, S., Charveron, M., Serre, G., & Simon, M. (2005). Peptidyl arginine deiminase isoforms 1–3 are expressed in the epidermis and involved in the deamination of K1 and filaggrin. *Journal of Investigative Dermatology, 124* (2), 384–393.

Nakazawa, D., Shida, H., Tomaru, U., Yoshida, M., Nishio, S., Atsumi, T., & Ishizu, A. (2014). Enhanced formation and disordered regulation of NETs in myeloperoxidase-ANCA-associated microscopic polyangiitis. *Journal of the American Society of Nephrology, 25*(12), 990–997. Available from https://doi.org/10.1681/ASN.2013060606.

Nakazawa, D., Tomaru, U., Suzuki, A., Masuda, S., Hasegawa, R., Kobayashi, T., ... Ishizu, A. (2012). Abnormal conformation and impaired degradation of propylthiouracil-induced neutrophil extracellular traps: Implications of disordered neutrophil extracellular traps in a rat model of myeloperoxidase antineutrophil cytoplasmic antibody-associated vasculiti. *Arthritis and Rheumatology, 64*(11), 3779–3787. Available from https://doi.org/10.1002/art.34619.

Nandi, B., & Behar, S. M. (2011). Regulation of neutrophils by interferon-gamma limits lung inflammation during tuberculosis infection. *Journal of Experimental Medicine, 208*(11), 2251–2262.

Nathan, C. (2006). Neutrophils and immunity: challenges and opportunities. *Nature Reviews Immunology, 6*, 173–182. Available from https://doi.org/10.1038/nri1785.

Neeli, I., Dwivedi, N., Khan, S., & Radic, M. (2009). Regulation of extracellular chromatin release from neutrophils. *Journal of Innate Immunity, 1*, 194−201. Available from https://doi.org/10.1159/000206974.

Nieminen, A., Maksimow, M., Mentula, P., Kyhälä, L., Kylänpää, L., Puolakkainen, P., ... Salmi, M. (2014). Circulating cytokines in predicting development of severe acute pancreatitis. *Critical Care, 18*(5), R104. Available from https://doi.org/10.1186/cc13885.

Olsson, A. K., & Cedervall, J. (2016). NETosis in cancer - platelet-neutrophil crosstalk promotes tumor-associated pathology. *Frontiers in Immunology, 7*, 373. Available from https://doi.org/10.3389/fimmu.2016.00373.

Pang, L., Hayes, C. P., Buac, K., Yoo, D. G., & Rada, B. (2013). Pseudogout-associated inflammatory calcium pyrophosphate dihydrate microcrystals induce formation of neutrophil extracellular traps. *Journal of Immunology, 190*(12), 6488−6500.

Papayannopoulos, V., Staab, D., & Zychlinsky, A. (2011). Neutrophil elastase enhances sputum solubilization in cystic fibrosis patients receiving dnase therapy. *PLoS One, 6*(12), e28526. Available from https://doi.org/10.1371/journal.pone.0028526.

Pertiwi, K. R., van der Wal, A. C., Pabittei, D. R., Mackaaij, C., van Leeuwen, M. B., & Li, X. (2018). Neutrophil extracellular traps participate in all different types of thrombotic and haemorrhagic complications of coronary atherosclerosis. *Thrombosis and Haemostasis, 118*(6), 1078−1087.

Pietronigro, E. C., Della Bianca, V., Zenaro, E., & Constantin, G. (2017). NETosis in Alzheimer's disease. *Frontiers in Immunology, 8*(211), 1−12. Available from https://doi.org/10.3389/fimmu.2017.00211.

Pillitteri, D., Bassus, S., Boller, K., Mahnel, R., Scholz, T., & Westrup, D. (2007). Thrombin-induced interleukin 1beta synthesis in platelet suspensions: Impact of contaminating leukocytes. *Platelets, 18*(2), 119−127. Available from https://doi.org/10.1080/09537100600800792.

Pilsczek, F. H., Salina, D., Poon, K. K., Fahey, C., Yipp, B. G., & Sibley, C. D. (2015). A novel mechanism of rapid nuclear neutrophil extracellular trap formation in response to Staphylococcus aureus. *Journal of Immunology, 185*, 7413−7425. Available from https://doi.org/10.4049/jimmunol.1000675.

Quan, J. M., Tiddens, H. A., Sy, J. P., McKenzie, S. G., Montgomery, M. D., Robinson, P. J., ... Pulmozyme Early Intervention Trial Study Group. (2001). A two-year randomized, placebo-controlled trial of dornase alfa in young patients with cystic fibrosis with mild lung function abnormalities. *Journal of Pediatrics, 139*(6), 813−820.

Querfurth, H. W., & LaFerla, F. M. (2010). Alzheimer's disease. *New England journal of medicine, 362*, 329−344. Available from https://doi.org/10.1056/NEJMra0909142.

Rada, B. (2017). Neutrophil extracellular trap release driven by bacterial motility: Relevance to cystic fibrosis lung disease. *Communicative and Integrative Biology, 10*(2), e1296610. Available from https://doi.org/10.1080/19420889.2017.1296610.

Rahman, S., & Gadjeva, M. (2014). Does NETosis contribute to the bacterial pathoadaptation in cystic fibrosis? *Frontiers in Immunology, 5*, 378. Available from https://doi.org/10.3389/fimmu.2014.00378.

Rodriguez-Espinosa, O., Rojas-Espinosa, O., Moreno-Altamirano, M. M., LopezVillegas, E. O., & Sanchez-Garcia, F. J. (2015). Metabolic requirements for neutrophil extracellular traps formation. *Immunology, 145*, 213−224. Available from https://doi.org/10.1111/imm.1243.

Rohrbach, A. S., Hemmers, S., Arandjelovic, S., Corr, M., & Mowen, K. A. (2012). PAD4 is not essential for disease in the K/BxN murine autoantibody-mediated model of arthritis. *Arthritis Research and Therapy, 14*(3), R104.

Rojek, L., Smoczynski, M., Stojek, M., Sledzinski, T., Smolenski, R. T., & Adrych, K. (2016). Increased protein degradation as well as lactate and malate dehydrogenase activity in sterile and infected walled-off pancreatic necrosis. *Polskie Archiwum Medycyny Wewnętrznej, 126* (3), 102−105. Available from https://doi.org/10.20452/pamw.3283.

Rossi, B., Angiari, S., Zenaro, E., Budui, S. L., & Constantin, G. (2011). Vascular inflammation in central nervous system diseases: Adhesion receptors controlling leukocyte-endothelial interactions. *Journal of Leukocyte Biology, 89*(4), 539−556. Available from https://doi.org/ 10.1189/jlb.0710432.

Saffarzadeh, M., Juenemann, C., Queisser, M. A., Lochnit, G., Barreto, G., Galuska, S. P., . . . Preissner, T. (2012). 'Neutrophil extracellular traps directly induce epithelial and endothelial cell death: A predominant role of histones. *PLoS One, 7*, e32366. Available from https://doi. org/10.1371/journal.pone.0032366.

Saitoh, T., Komano, J., Saitoh, Y., Misawa, T., Takahama, M., Kozaki, T., . . . Akira, S. (2012). Neutrophil extracellular traps mediate a host defense response to human immunodeficiency virus-1. *Cell Host Microbe, 12*(1), 109−116. Available from https://doi.org/10.1016/j. chom.2012.05.015.

Sica, A., Schioppa, T., Mantovani, A., & Allavena, P. (2006). Tumour-associated macrophages are a distinct M2 polarised population promoting tumour progression: Potential targets of anti-cancer therapy. *European Journal of Cancer, 42*(6), 717−727. Available from https:// doi.org/10.1016/j.ejca.2006.01.003.

Sil, P., Hayes, C. P., Reaves, B. J., Breen, P., Quinn, S., Sokolove, J., & Rada, B. (2016). P2Y6 receptor antagonist MRS2578 inhibits neutrophil activation and aggregated neutrophil extra-cellular trap formation induced by gout-associated monosodium urate crystals. *The Journal of Immunology, 198*(1), 428−442. Available from https://doi.org/10.4049/jimmunol.1600766.

Skopelja, S., Hamilton, B. J., Jones, J. D., Yang, M. L., Mamula, M., Ashare, A., . . . Rigby, W. F. (2016). The role for neutrophil extracellular traps in cystic fibrosis autoimmunity. *JCI Insight, 1*(1), e88912.

Sollberger, G., Tilley, D. O., & Zychlinsky, A. (2018). Neutrophil extracellular traps: The biol-ogy of chromatin externalization. *Developmental Cell, 44*(5), 542−553.

Springer, D. J., Ren, P., Raina, R., Dong, Y., Behr, M. J., & McEwen, B. F. (2010). Extracellular fibrils of pathogenic yeast *Cryptococcus gattii* are important for ecological niche, murine virulence and human neutrophil interactions. *PLoS One, 5*(6), e10978. Available from https://doi.org/10.1371/journal.pone.0010978.

Tarkowski, E., Andreasen, N., Tarkowski, A., & Blennow, K. (2003). Intrathecal inflammation precedes development of Alzheimer's disease. *Journal of Neurology, Neurosurgery, and Psychiatry, 74*(9), 1200−1205. Available from https://doi.org/10.1136/jnnp.74.9.1200.

Tenner, S., Baillie, J., DeWitt, J., & Vege, S. S. (2013). American College of Gastroenterology guideline: management of acute pancreatitis. *American Journal of Gastroenterology, 108*(9), 1400−1415. Available from https://doi.org/10.1038/ajg.2013.218.

Tomson, A. H. (1995). Human recombinant DNase in cystic fibrosis. *Journal of Royal Society of Medicine, 88*(Suppl 25), 24−29.

Tong, L., Chi, C., & Zhang, Z. (2018). Association of various glycemic variability indices and vascular outcomes in type-2 diabetes patients: A retrospective study. *Medicine, 97*(21), e10860. Available from https://doi.org/10.1097/MD.0000000000010860.

Ueno, A., Murakami, K., Yamanouchi, K., Watanabe, M., & Kondo, T. (1996). Thrombin stimu-lates production of interleukin-8 in human umbilical vein endothelial cells. *Immunology, 88* (1), 76−81.

Urban, C. F., Reichard, U., Brinkmann, V., & Zychlinsky, A. (2006). Neutrophil extracellular traps capture and kill *Candida albicans* yeast and hyphal forms. *Cellular Microbiology*, *8*(4), 668−676. Available from https://doi.org/10.1111/j.1462-5822.2005.00659.x.

von Brühl, M. L., Stark, K., Steinhart, A., Chandraratne, S., Konrad, I., Lorenz, M., . . . Massberg, S. (2012). Monocytes, neutrophils, and platelets cooperate to initiate and propagate venous thrombosis in mice in vivo. *Journal of Experimental Medicine*, *209*(4), 819−835. Available from https://doi.org/10.1084/jem.20112322.

Vukic, V., Callaghan, D., Walker, D., Lue, L. F., Liu, Q. Y., Couraud, P. O., . . . Zhang, W. (2009). Expression of inflammatory genes induced by beta-amyloid peptides in human brain endothelial cells and in Alzheimer's brain is mediated by the JNK-AP1 signaling pathway. *Neurobiology of Disease*, *34*(1), 95−106. Available from https://doi.org/10.1016/j.nbd.2008.12.007.

Wall, I., Badalov, N., Baradarian, R., Iswara, K., Li, J. J., & Tenner, S. (2011). Decreased mortality in acute pancreatitis related to early aggressive hydration. *Pancreas*, *40*(4), 547−550. Available from https://doi.org/10.1097/MPA.0b013e318215368d.

Wang, W., Wang, Y., Long, J., Wang, J., Haudek, S. B., Overbeek, P., . . . Danesh, F. R. (2012). Mitochondrial fission triggered by hyperglycemia is mediated by ROCK1 activation in podocytes and endothelial cells. *Cell Metabolism*, *15*(2), 186−200.

Warnatsch, A., Ioannou, M., Wang, Q., & Papayannopoulos, V. (2015). Inflammation. Neutrophil extracellular traps license macrophages for cytokine production in atherosclerosis. *Science*, *349*(6245), 316−320.

Wei, F., Sun, X., Zhao, Y., Zhang, H., Diao, Y., & Liu, Z. (2016). Excessive visit-to-visit glycemic variability independently deteriorates the progression of endothelial and renal dysfunction in patients with type 2 diabetes mellitus. *Bio Med Central Nephrology*, *17*, 67.

Werner, J., Hartwig, W., Hackert, T., Kaiser, H., Schmidt, J., Gebhard, M. M., . . . Klar, E. (2012). Multidrug strategies are effective in the treatment of severe experimental pancreatitis. *Surgery*, *151*(3), 372−381.

Wong, S. L., Demers, M., Martinod, K., Gallant, M., Wang, Y., Goldfne, A. B., . . . Wagner, D. D. (2015). Diabetes primes neutrophils to undergo NETosis, which impairs wound healing. *Nature Medicine*, *21*(7), 815−819. Available from https://doi.org/10.1038/nm.3887.

Yamagishi, S., Nakamura, N., Suematsu, M., Kaseda, K., & Matsui, T. (2015). Advanced glycation end products: a molecular target for vascular complications in diabetes. *Molecular Medicine*, *21*(Suppl 1), S32−S40. Available from https://doi.org/10.2119/molmed.2015.00067.

Yamamoto, K., Yamada, H., Wakana, N., Kikai, M., Terada, K., Wada, N., . . . Matoba, S. (2018). Augmented neutrophil extracellular traps formation promotes atherosclerosis development in socially defeated apoE-/- mice. *Biochemical and Biophysical Research Communications*, *500*(2), 490−496.

Yin, X., Wright, J., Wall, T., & Grammas, P. (2010). Brain endothelial cells synthesize neurotoxic thrombin in Alzheimer's disease. *The American Journal of Pathology*, *176*(4), 1600−1606. Available from https://doi.org/10.2353/ajpath.2010.090406.

Yoo, D., Floyd, M., Winn, M., Moskowitz, S. M., & Rada, B. (2014). NET formation induced by *Pseudomonas aeruginosa* cystic fibrosis isolates measured as release of myeloperoxidase−DNA and neutrophil elastase−DNA complexes. *Immunology Letters*, *160*(2), 186−194.

Young, R. L., Malcolm, K. C., Kret, J. E., Caceres, S. M., Poch, K. R., Nichols, D. P., . . . Nick, J. A. (2011). Neutrophil extracellular trap (NET)-mediated killing of *Pseudomonas Aeruginosa*: Evidence of acquired resistance within the CF airway, independent of CFTR. *PLoS One*, *6*(9), e23637.

Zawrotniak, M., & Rapala-Kozik, M. (2013). Neutrophil extracellular traps (NETs) - formation and implications. *Acta Biochimica Polonica, 60*(3), 277−284.

Zenaro, E., Piacentino, G., & Constantin, G. (2017). The blood-brain barrier in Alzheimer's disease. *Neurobiology of Disease, 107,* 41−56. Available from https://doi.org/10.1016/j.nbd.2016.07.007.

Zenaro, E., Pietronigro, E., Della Bianca, V., Piacentino, G., Marongiu, L., Budui, S., ... Constantin, G. (2015). Neutrophils promote Alzheimer's disease-like pathology and cognitive decline via LFA-1 integrin. *Nature Medicine, 21*(8), 880−886. Available from https://doi.org/10.1038/nm.3913.

Zhang, S., Lu, X., Shu, X., Tian, X., Yang, H., Yang, W., ... Wang, G. (2014). Elevated plasma cfDNA may be associated with active lupus nephritis and partially attributed to abnormal regulation of neutrophil extracellular traps (NETs) in patients with systemic lupus erythematosus. *Internal Medicine, 53*(24), 2763−2771. Available from https://doi.org/10.2169/internalmedicine.53.2570.

Zhao, W., Fogg, D. K., & Kaplan, M. J. (2015). A novel image-based quantitative method for the characterization of NETosis. *Journal of Immunological Methods, 423,* 104−110. Available from https://doi.org/10.1016/j.jim.2015.04.027.

Zhu, L., Kuang, Z., Wilson, B. A., & Lau, G. W. (2013). Competence-independent activity of pneumococcal EndA [corrected] mediates degradation of extracellular DNA and nets and is important for virulence. *PLoS One, 8,* e70363. Available from https://doi.org/10.1371/journal.pone.0070363.

Zlokovic, B. V. (2011). Neurovascular pathways to neurodegeneration in Alzheimer's disease and other disorders. *Nature Reviews Neuroscience, 12*(12), 723−738. Available from https://doi.org/10.1038/nrn3114.

Further reading

Menegazzo, L., Scattolini, V., Cappellari, R., Bonora, B. M., Albiero, M., Bortolozzi, M., ... Fadini, G. P. (2018). The antidiabetic drug metformin blunts NETosis in vitro and reduces circulating NETosis biomarkers in vivo. *Acta Diabetologica, 55*(6), 593−601. Available from https://doi.org/10.1007/s00592-018-1129-8.

Nomenclature list

μm	micrometer
A1AT	alpha 1-antitrypsin
AA	adjuvant-induced arthritis
AAV	ANCA-associated vasculitis
ACPAs	anticitrullinated protein antibodies
ADP	adenosine diphosphate
AggNETs	aggregated NETs
AMP	antimicrobial peptide
ANAs	antinuclear autoantibodies
ANCA	antineutrophil cytoplasmic antibodies
Apaf1	apoptotic protease activating factor
APCs	antigen presenting cells
ATG7	autophagy-related protein 7
ATP	adenosine triphosphate
AVOs	acidic vesicular organelles
AZU1	azurocidin 1
BAFF	B cell activating factor
BCP	basic calcium phosphate
BET	basophil extracellular traps
BLM	belimumab
BPI	bactericidal permeability increasing protein
CAD	caspase-activated DNase
CARM1	coactivator associated arginine methyltransferase 1
CCR5	C−C chemokine receptor type 5
CD	Crohn's disease
CD4	cluster of differentiation 4
CDK	cyclin dependent kinases
cfDNA	cell free DNA
CFTR	cystic fibrosis transmembrane regulator
CGD	chronic granulomatous disease
CitH3	histone citrullination
CNS	central nervous system
COPD	chronic obstructive pulmonary disease
CPPD	calcium pyrophosphate dehydrate crystals
CR3	complement receptor 3
CRISSP	cancer associated SCM recognition, immune defense suppression and serine protease protection peptide
CTSC	cathepsin C

CXCR	C-X-C motif chemokine receptor
DAMP	damage-associated molecular patterns
DCs	dendritic cells
DENV	dengue virus
DISC	death-inducing signaling complex
DN	double negative
DPI	diphenylene iodonium
dsDNA	double stranded DNA
EBNA	Epstein–Barr nuclear antigen
ECP	eosinophil cationic protein
EET	eosinophil extracellular traps
ELANE	elastase, neutrophil-expressed
ELISA	enzyme linked immunosorbent assay
ELS	ectopic lymphoid structures
ER	endoplasmic reticulum
ERK	extracellular-signal-regulated kinase
FADD	Fas-associated protein with death domain
FCγRI	Fc gamma receptor 1
FDC	follicular dendritic cells
fMLP	formyl-methionyl-leucyl-phenylalanine
Fn	fibronectin
FPR	formyl-peptide receptors
G-CSF	granulocyte colony-stimulating factor
GC	germinal center
GDP	guanosine diphosphate
GEFs	guanine nucleotide exchange factors
GM-CSF	granulocyte/macrophage colony-stimulating factor
GSDMD	gasdermin D
GTP	guanosine triphosphate
GXM	glucuronoxylomannan
H3R26	histone h3 arginine26
HCO₃	bicarbonate
HEVs	high endothelial venules
HIF	hypoxia-inducible factor
HIV 1	human immunodeficiency virus 1
HLA-Dr	human leukocyte antigen—Dr isotype
HMGB 1	high mobility group box 1
HNP	human neutrophil peptide
HOCl	hypochlorous acid
HSP	heat shock protein
HUVEC	human umbilical vein endothelial cells
IFN	interferon
Ig	immunoglobulin
IL	interleukin
IRAK	IL-1 receptor-associated kinase
IRS	insulin receptor substrate
JAK	Janus kinase

LC	light chain
LCP1	lymphocyte cytosolic protein 1
LDGs	low density granulocytes
LFA 1	lymphocyte function associated antigen 1
LPS	lipopolysaccharide
Luk GH	leukotoxin GH
MAC	membrane attack complex
MAPK	microtubule associated protein kinase
MBP	major basic protein
MCET	mast cell extracellular traps
MEK	MAPK/ERK kinase
mitoROS	mitochondrial reactive oxygen species
MLKL	mixed lineage kinase domain like protein
MMPs	matrix metalloproteases
MODS	multiple organ dysfunction syndrome
MPO	myeloperoxidase
MROS	mitochondrial reactive oxygen species
Ms	multiple sclerosis
MSU	monosodium urate
mtDNA	mitochondrial DNA
mTOR	mammalian target of rapamycin
MYH9	myosin 9
Myo1C	myosin 1C
NA	not applicable
NaCl	sodium chloride
NADPH	nicotinamide adenine dinucleotide phosphate hydrolase
ND	not determined
NE	neutrophil elastase
NEC	necrotizing enterocolitis
NET	neutrophil extracellular trap
NF	nuclear factor
NF κB	nuclear factor kappa B
NLR	NOD-like receptors
NLRP3	NOD, LRR, and pyrin domain containing 3
nm	nanometer
nNIF	neonatal NET inhibitory factor
NO	nitric oxide
NOD	nucleotide binding and oligomerization domain
NOX	NADPH oxidase
NPs	nanoparticles
NRPs	net related peptides
NZM	New Zealand mixed 2328 (model of murine lupus)
O_2	oxygen
OD	organ dysfunction
OLFM4	olfactomedin 4
PAD	peptidyl arginine deiminase
PAF	platelet activating factor
Paks	P-21 activated kinases
PAMP	pathogen-associated molecular patterns

PDCs	plasma dendritic cells
pH$_e$	extracellular pH
pH$_i$	intracellular pH
PHOX	phagocytic oxidase
PI3K	phosphoinositide 3-kinase
PKC	protein kinase C
PMA	phorbol-12 myristate13-acetate
PMNs	polymorphonuclear neutrophils
PR	proteinase
PRMT1	protein arginine methyltransferase 1
PRR	pattern-recognizing receptors
PSGL 1	P-selectin glycoprotein ligand 1
PTPN22	protein tyrosin phospatase
PVL	Panton–Valentine leucocidin
RA	rheumatoid arthritis
Raf	rapidly accelerated fibrosarcoma
RAGE	receptor for advanced glycation end products
rhDNase	recombinant human DNase
RIPK	receptor interacting serine/threonine protein kinase
ROS	reactive oxygen species
RRMS	relapsing remitting multiple sclerosis
RSV	respiratory syncytial virus
RTX	rituximab
SCM	squamous cell metaplasia
SEs	shared epitopes
SIRL1	signal inhibitory receptor on leukocytes 1
SK3	small conductance calcium-activated potassium channel protein 3
SLE	systemic lupus erythematosus
SMA	small urate microaggregates
SNP	single nucleotide polymorphisms
SOD	superoxide dismutase
SS	Sjögren's syndrome
T2DM	type 2 diabetes mellitus
TCZ	tocilizumab
TF	tissue factor
THAM	tris hydroxymethyl aminomethane, tromethamine
THP	Tamm–Horsfall protein
TIMPs	tissue inhibitors of metalloproteinases
TLR	toll like receptor
TNF	tumor necrosis factor
TNFR	tumor necrosis factor receptor
TP	triptolide
TRALI	transfusion-related acute lung injury
TUNEL	terminal deoxynucleotidyl transferase
UC	ulcerative colitis
UV	ultraviolet

Index

Note: Page numbers followed by "*f*" and "*t*" refer to figures and tables, respectively.

Printed in the United States
By Bookmasters